UNDERSTANDING CANCER

UNDERSTANDING CANCER

Bryan N. Brooke

HOLT, RINEHART AND WINSTON
NEW YORK   CHICAGO   SAN FRANCISCO

Contents

44586

Preface

For too long doctors have been jealous of the treasure they possess – the knowledge, as far as it goes, of how man behaves and how his body works in health and in disorder. The attitude is changing for the knowledge is fascinating to all; moreover we all have a right to know about ourselves.

Difficulties arise in setting the scene for cancer, for while this book may be of some interest to those with inside knowledge it is written for those who have not. To understand cancer requires a modicum of biological knowledge; it also needs a passing acquaintance with unfamiliar terms and words. I have endeavoured to overcome these difficulties by gradual explanation and avoidance, as far as possible, of technical terms. My family, with much patience to which I wish to pay tribute, have read, queried and corrected for me; they are quite innocent of medical terms since 'shop' is strictly forbidden in the home. The outcome, I hope, is a book which can be read and understood by anyone including those who have had the misfortune to be deprived of even a smattering of biology at school. Whenever a new concept or word has arisen for the first time it has been explained. However, I know only too well how difficult it is to retain clearly in one's mind the meaning of a new and unfamiliar word. To assist recall a brief glossary has therefore been included at the end. It is my hope that most readers will find no need for recourse to this.

B.N.B.

CHAPTER ONE

Introduction

Doctors have been so secretive about their affairs, about disease and its effects but are now less uncommunicative. This attitude in the past needs some explanation. It was dictated by conventions which reach back in time to an era when medicine was conducted on the charitable basis of the voluntary hospital, when education was not universal, when those who were educated had no part in science: so that explanation was usually impossible, was not expected and very unlikely to be proffered. Fear of death and the concept of incurability made a virtue of secrecy for it was clearly bad for the patient to know, though it might be wise to inform the relations who were thus drawn into the collusion of secrecy. The virtue, thus hallowed, became converted into the phenomenon of a taboo eminently suitable for anthropological study. For the doctor, this virtue coincided with the ordinary frailty to be expected of a human: for who would welcome the task of informing the patient of the implication of his disease? Most of us can summon the strength for a distasteful task but to appear to don the black cap and condemn is not within us. Thankfully, social mores allowed us to make a virtue of secrecy, a virtue of non-disclosure and the avoidance of a cruel, hateful task. It became our responsibility not to tell, to indulge in circumvention and to maintain the white lie.

   We can no longer resort to subterfuge and many no longer do, for time, the evolution of science, its communication to all and its comprehension by almost all, the very spread of rationality pervading our community, have evoked great change. Nevertheless, certain taboos remain. Sex is off the list though clearly in the phase of aftermath and overswing. But the taboos about death, cancer and even pain remain. All require the exposure of understanding and rational appreciation and this will doubtless happen as the civilizing influences of our social life continue to develop.

Cancer is still subject to considerable taboo; the impression, albeit erroneous, that its *alter ego* is death has linked and fortified the taboos, as indeed has the equally erroneous supposition that cancer is synonymous with pain. Indeed a moment's reflection will reveal that pain is not an invariable feature of cancer for the disease is usually insidious in onset and could not be so if pain were dominant. It is odd, too, that the identification between cancer and death is so strong in people's minds. That cancer is often deadly is incontrovertible, but the range of malignancy covered by cancer is so wide that many varieties are not so. The degree of malignancy is infinitely variable and even the more malignant types do not compare either in deadliness, disability or distress, with other common disorders – arterial disease for example – which are freely discussed and frequently without a shudder. Though the considerable therapeutic effort, skill and determination applied to malignancy is often ineffectual, the natural history of this state equally often displays slow development so that the outcome, undeflected by treatment, can still be less disastrous and less handicapping than other disorders we are prepared to contemplate and openly discuss.

The truth is that cancer is an emotive word invoking superstition, suggesting a sinister attack from a wicked mystery outside ourselves. It is hardly seen as a biological change, a failure of cell mechanics. Fear and superstition should have been released by knowledge yet their thraldom remains because the emotive force reflected in and reinforced by the imagery conveyed by the very word, cancer, holds public and doctors alike in the convention of silence. Post-war trends have revealed the beginnings of awareness by doctors that medical knowledge is not their prerogative alone, that patients have a right to know about themselves and about the implications of disease when it assails them. The avidity of the public for medical knowledge is obvious. No evidence is forthcoming that access to medical information increases fear, neuroticism, depression or panic, objections given in the past by doctors, who seem not to have observed that they are no more afflicted themselves by these emotions when they fall sick, despite their special knowledge – and nobody could argue that doctors have a special dispensation of fortitude above the average.

The taboo about cancer should now be laid. It may be incurable; but so are many other common diseases which nevertheless are considered, contemplated and understood by all. But life itself is an incurable disorder in that it must end in death. And not so rarely, cancer itself is overtaken by another disorder and beaten to the final post.

CHAPTER TWO

The Nature of Cancer

Some knowledge of the structure of the human body is needed if cancer is to be understood at all, not so much in the sense of where different organs lie and their relationship to one another but how any part is constructed. Everything is based on the cell, the brick from which is built the whole unit, be it an organ such as the liver, kidney, lung and brain, or a tissue such as muscle or bone. A cell is in fact the lowest common denominator of living things beyond which we cannot go in terms of life. Groups of cells may become separated from their fellows and yet persist but continuous activity will cease if cell structure itself is lost.

Looked at through a microscope this unit of life is composed of a dense central core, the nucleus, floating in a clearer substance, the cytoplasm, all being held together in a thin envelope, the cell membrane. The shape and size of cells vary from organ to organ and are distinguishable so that it is possible to recognize through the microscope which organ they belong to. Function of the part dictates the shape of its cell. Muscle being a tissue which contracts needs elongated strands interlacing with one another rather as a strand of wool is built up from the hairs of a fleece. A nerve cell outside the brain is very long and thin for it is analogous to a telephone wire. In organs which secrete fluids, such as the kidney, or tissues like the lining of stomach and intestine where digestive juices are prepared, the cells are more compact. They are square or rectangular because they lie cheek by jowl in tiers. When cells are stuck together in larger masses they begin to appear hexagonal or octagonal due to their more numerous juxtapositions.

Within the blood which is not only fluid but contains red cells to carry oxygen and white cells to protect the body from harmful intrusion of any sort, the cells are circular. They have to flow with the blood stream and roll along its innumerable channels. In fact the red cells are circular discs indented on their flat surfaces. This gives various advantages. The concavity increases the surface area thus facilitating the exchange of oxygen between the special compound for oxygen transport, the haemoglobin, inside and the tissue outside. Being flat many cells can be packed together in the ducting system; if the cells were completely round oxygen diffusion would be slower and each component of oxygen carrying power would take up more room. The white cells are round since their function makes no such demands of physical transfer. They engulf bacteria or create chemicals, antibodies and antitoxins, to counter the effects of bacteria or indeed any noxious chemical which may find its way into the body system.

In the lungs oxygen has to be passed from the air to the red cell. At the same time the blood must be contained; obviously it cannot lie free in a pool of air. So the lining of the lungs is made up of many chambers, called alveoli, all connected through the bronchial tubes to the main wind-pipe, the trachea. Between the walls of each alveolus run the tiny thin vessels containing the blood. The cells which form the alveolar walls are therefore very thin so that oxygen may easily pass through into the blood. They are also elastic, for recoil is necessary to drive out the used air in the chamber on expiration. Their shape and size therefore vary just as a muscle cell must do as it contracts.

Whatever the task the cell structure remains the same –

a membrane to contain the cytoplasm in which floats the nucleus – with one exception. The mature red cell carries no nucleus. It does not need to for only a sac is required to carry haemoglobin, the chemical with the peculiar ability of giving up oxygen to tissues where required and taking it on again rapidly in the lung. A nucleus is present in the cell as it is developed in the bone marrow but this is shed on maturity and the cell starts its three-week-long life in the blood stream. It then needs no nucleus for unlike other cells it has no independent activity once it is launched; nor does it have to reproduce itself, for red cells are prepared from nucleated parent cells in the bone marrow.

Anyone who has had the opportunity to look at botanical or biological specimens under a microscope will be familiar with these appearances and will carry in their mind's eye an idea of the size of an average cell. With the exception of the ovum which varies greatly throughout the animal kingdom, the somatic, that is the body cells, are much the same in girth and length tissue for tissue from one species to another. At microscopic levels measurement is registered in microns, 1 micron being one millionth part of a metre. The red cell seen side on is 2 microns thick and 8 microns in diameter viewed from in front. Of the white blood cells the lymphocyte, which becomes very important in our story later, is about the same size but is spherical. Other white cells, less important to the subject of cancer so that we do not need to consider them in detail, are a little larger from 9–12 microns, sufficiently large in fact to be distinguishable under the microscope from lymphocytes. In terms of microns the range of other cells is quite wide, as is their shape.

Epithelial cells, those that form the surface to skin, gut, lung and urinary tract for instance, vary according to function. As already stated those which line the alveoli in

6

the lungs are thin to permit the ready diffusion of oxygen into the blood. In the gut the epithelium has a secretory function so the cells are bigger and fatter, being square or rectangular in cross-section, forming, as in the lung, a layer one cell thick. By contrast the epithelium of the skin produces a covering several cells in depth and as the surface is reached they loose their nuclei becoming just horny scales to keep out the wet and keep in the tissue fluid – waterproofing both ways. Some of the skin cells become specialized so that they can secrete sweat and sebum, the oily film which maintains texture and also helps to prevent us drying out.

Muscle cells are very different and nobody knows quite how long they can be, for while a muscle cell may be anything from 10 to 100 microns in girth, it can extend in length to over 100 millimetres, possibly more. And nerves have a main cell body from which wirelike filaments emerge some of which may be extremely long where connection has to be made from the spinal cord into a limb, for instance.

Size and shape of cells is determined therefore, as is only reasonable, by function. These forms gradually become manifest as each tissue is developed in the embryo, each becoming differentiated from the other starting from a round totipotential cell, the ovum. How one tissue gains its distinction from another we shall see shortly.

So far we have been concerned only with the appearances of cells, their morphology. This is less important than how they work. Every cell is a basic particle of some specific tissue and is specific to that tissue. A liver cell is a liver cell is a liver cell – to plagiarize Stein – and it cannot switch to become something else. It has one function, or set of functions, relevant to the organ to which it belongs. A liver cell cannot suddenly switch and function as though it were in the kidney. Moreover, though the liver cell may not look very different from one in the kidney, the results they achieve are very different, as different as the chemist from the plumber. Each cell is a most exact dynamic structure equipped to provide a function appropriate to its place wherever that may be.

The key to cell function lies in the nucleus, that dense central material. This is the jig, the former plate which sets the repetitive task; it even makes what adjustments may be necessary both in the quality and volume of work the cell does. It also stamps the cell with its identity not only in terms of the work it does but also by ensuring that it will replace itself by an exactly similar cell for, except in the nervous system and to some extent muscle, cells are finite; they cannot live as long as the individual. So the nucleus dictates the work and ensures its own replacement.

In lonely company with the muscle cells of the heart, nerve cells last a lifetime in the brain and in the nerves which lead from and to it in order to provide intelligence and communication. If a nerve cell is destroyed by disease it cannot be replaced, though the long wire, the neurone, which leads from the cell can grow out again after it has been cut provided the rest of the cell and its nucleus are intact. Similarly heart muscle cannot replace itself. In coronary thrombosis an area of heart muscle is destroyed. It is only patched up by scar tissue, for the cells of the heart like nerve cannot replicate.

The nucleus is of vital importance – literally. It is a complex substance deposited as a long filament coiled up like a wormcast. It contains molecules of special materials called desoxyribonucleic (D.N.A.) and ribonucleic acids (R.N.A.). The former stamps the cell with its identity – what tissue it is part of and what species it belongs to – so that it can certainly reproduce itself in exactly similar form. It also dictates the work to be done and this is carried

8

out by the R.N.A. Though the same material, D.N.A., is used throughout the animal kingdom for creating the cell nucleus, nevertheless the nuclei differ from species to species so that separate and specific identity is obtained. Thus a liver cell in mouse would not be like that in man. This is achieved by different quantities of protein and D.N.A., and different arrangement of the D.N.A. molecular chain.

In order to reproduce itself the coiled chain unfolds itself and breaks into separate links, called chromosomes, which then split longitudinally so that two sets of chromosomes, each the image of the other, is produced. The whole cell can then divide and the next cell-generation is born. Each species has a fixed number of chromosomes; man has 46. So every cell throughout man's body wherever it may be has a nucleus coded as man by the possession of 46 chromosomes. Again there is a subdivision: for the chromosomes, comprised as they are of protein and D.N.A. molecules, carry the genes and it is these which dictate the individual's characteristics – whether his eyes are blue, his hair red and so on. Genes are the lesser parts of chromosomes, linked together yet distinguished by their place on the chromosome filament and by the arrangement of certain small simpler chemicals stuck to them. An infinite variety of pattern is thus obtained to provide the template which sets the cell identity and the task it has to perform. This will be clear to those who have read that exciting book the *Double Helix*.

The R.N.A. moiety of the nucleus simply organizes the work of the cell under the direction of its D.N.A.; it has no part in cell identity so necessary for cell reproduction. It ensures that a cell implicated for example in producing a secretion creates molecules of the correct substance from the various materials at its disposal in the cell cytoplasm; that these are passed along the ducting system which provides the communication network within the cell (called the endoplasmic reticulum) and eventually out into the secretory ducts which drain the material away from the cell to the site where it is to be used. Thus some cells in the lining of the stomach produce hydrochloric acid and others a digestive enzyme called pepsin; both substances are poured down little drains around which these cells are clustered, into the stomach where they can be mixed with food by the churning movements of the muscle of the stomach wall.

So each tissue begets itself – with the exception of nerves and heart muscle. What has not been explained is how tissue specificity is obtained in the process of development. We start life as one cell, the fertilized ovum. That cell has one nucleus and contained within that one nucleus is the extraordinary potential of producing a multitude of different cell-lines each differentiated from other cell-lines to create all the multifarious tissues of the adult body. Nobody has explained how the original nuclear pattern in the ovum carries so many different templates for the future adult; nor how at a given moment of embryonic life in the womb the three basic embryonic tissues which are the next stage forward from the ovum sprout their new and different fledglings, each to provide new tissues for our separate organs.

The ovum divides into two, then into four and so on until a solid mass becomes a hollow balloon. Almost as soon as this appears it disappears being indented, as though the balloon were pricked and one wall invaginated into the other. From the inner layer, called the endoderm, all lining cells for the gut are derived. It is not, of course, so different from the outer layer, the ectoderm, which provides skin and the linings of organs such as the bladder and the pipes running to and from it. Between these two lies a middle layer of cells, the mesoderm which gives rise to muscle, bone, supporting tissue and blood. This early differentiation has some relevance to our story for cancer is prone to occur in those tissues which had their origin in ecto- and endo-derm. With the exception of the white cells of the blood, cancer is uncommon in tissue of meso-dermal origin.

At certain predestined stages of growth in the womb one organ after another appears so that the foetus begins to become recognizable as a human form, or at least as a hominid. But nobody knows how the nuclei of the early undifferentiated cells switch on to new cell-lines nor how the right moment for change and deployment is dictated. A time element is built in; a rhythmicity of cell activity, which may be an intrinsic feature of complex protein molecules, could be the answer. We just do not know, though it begins to appear that chains of protein mole-cules are intrinsically capable of increasing by continu-ously budding out more molecules. Thus nucleoprotein goes on growing in length, divides and grows again.

The complexity required in each cell nucleus to register what species it belongs to and what function it must undertake contains yet another factor. Just as each person is an individual distinguishable from another, so are his cells. His cells carry the special genetic structure which give him his individuality, the colour of his hair, the shape of his body, his very temperament. And all this comes from his parents, not wholly from one nor wholly from the other, but an admixture from each through the ovum and sperm, each of which carry half the nuclear material of any mature cell.

The chromosomes in a nucleus are all paired. So for man we should think not of 46 chromosomes but 23 pairs. On one pair is registered the individual's sex; the other 22, called autosomes, carry every other function – a slight oversimplification, since the sex chromosomes carry some other functions but it is this pair which determines the sex. In each autosomal pair the chromosomes are identical. Only in the sex chromosomes are the pair unlike and then only in the male. The female chromosome is conventionally labelled X and the male Y. A woman carries the female pair, XX, but a man is not, as you might suppose, YY but XY. YY is, in fact, incompatible with life.

To achieve the reduction of nuclear material necessary for sperm or ovum all that has to occur is separation of the pairs. In ordinary cell division which we considered earlier the chromosomal pairs divide into two paired sets. In cell division to create the reproductive unit the pairs separate instead of dividing. So all ova contain 23 single chromosomes, one of which is X. Sperms also possess 23 single chromosomes but with a 50–50 chance of X or Y in each set. So each gamete (that is an ovum or a sperm) has 23 chromosomes and when fusion between the two occurs the normal pairing is restored.

What develops from this fusion, from the fertilized ovum in effect, will depend upon the admixture of genes and chromosomes from two individuals. It is a strange thought that human cells have an immortality denied to their host, for human cell-lines are carried unchanged within the individual and across in part to the next generation. It is only at this stage that there is opportunity for change within the species. Thus you are unlike, or only partially like, your parents; biological change ebbs and flows to and fro across generations of men. But each individual is set in his image. Once born there is no chance, so long as you remain normal, that the form of your tissues will change. The liver will remain the liver, the characteristics which identify the individual as a person will remain. However, normality is a wholly theoretical concept.

So why do we not go on for ever, just as we were when

we became full grown? Because, like all automatic processes, from time to time something goes wrong – though
to use the word 'wrong' begs the question of life, which is
in essence change. The nucleus is not immutable; nuclear
division for replication or reproduction does not always
go smoothly. It may split unevenly passing to the next
generation of cells more chromosomes or more substance
of a chromosome, or less, and a new line of cells is formed,
which will behave differently because the template has
changed. The new cell-line may wither away so no harm
is done – that is, no abnormal function may develop. Or
the new line is so infinitesimally small in number compared with the total mass of cells belonging to that tissue
that they do not make their presence felt. Not at first: not
at all, if they do not survive. But if they do, gradually from
the one cell of altered replication grow many others to
provide a change in function of the part as their impact
causes the original form to yield in competition. Thus disorder becomes manifest as change within change. For life
is change, the vast flowing biochemical change of the
second by second activity derived from innumerable cells
in proper form, as predictable as the seasons or diurnal
variation. But even the solstices begin to vary with disorder.

The nucleus is not inviolate. Protein can react with protein, can attach itself to protein; they only have to make
contact. The cell wall, designed to permit molecules not
too large and not too complex through its portcullis, will
jib at complex protein, simply because the molecule is too
bulky, too angular, too generally cumbersome to make
the passage. But the wall can be battered or pierced; the
membrane succumbs to certain protein endowed with the
power of penetration by its actual shape – the virus. Not
all viruses have this power but once within the cell some
viruses can attach themselves to the nuclear protein or

actually take over from it. A new nucleo-protein, the viral template, then orders the activity of the cell to its own design and that order is disorder to man.

Minute fast-moving particles can penetrate the cell, as does meteoric dust the spaceship wall – gamma rays, X-rays, even the cosmic dust, the neutrons which have previously succeeded in passing through the earth's atmospheric shield. Protein comprising the nucleus is a delicate structure easily shattered by a hit; the template changes; the cell function stops if mutilation is too great but the altered cell may persist and be left with one function – just the ability to reproduce itself, replication is the exact word. And that is cancer.

Moreover, the cancer cell can pursue this single purpose of replication almost without let or hindrance. Normal cells are kept in control in this respect. If you lose part of your liver by disease or accident, the normal liver cells which remain increase their rate of reproduction so as to fill the gap. Once this is filled, the rate drops to what is required to maintain ordinary cell turnover to replace wear and tear; otherwise the liver would get bigger and bigger. How this control is brought about remains unknown, but clearly an impossible situation would arise if organs continued to increase in size regardless of other organs and the body economy generally. Some fluctuation indeed does take place in response to the dictates of the moment – of special demands arising from the body's function. Thus muscle masses will increase in response to physical exertion. The thyroid increases each month in menstruating women because of an increased metabolic demand at such a time and the thyroid controls the rate at which we burn up our fuel – all part of metabolism.

But this process never goes too far; it is all under control and serves the total needs of the body. Not so with the cancer cell; it has its own anarchic autonomy. It is so perversely maverick that the cells never get together to produce an organized whole in recognizable form so that an organ can be distinguished. The cells lie side by side haphazardly in an amorphous mass which shows none of the self-restraint of normal cells, contact inhibition as it is called. They may only be constrained by the immunological defences inherent in the lymphocytes.

Though a tendency towards cancerous change appears in some families the cancer nucleus itself is not imparted from one generation to another. In familial cancer a genetic defect may be carried in the original cell; this defect then causes the cells of certain tissues later to change so that in some a cancer nucleus develops. There is a rare example of this affecting the intestine. A genetic tendency is inherited which follows clearly a recognizable genetic pattern known as Mendelian dominance. Cancer does not appear at birth in affected members of such a family; as time passes, as long as twenty years or more, cancer begins to be seen in the lining of the large intestine. It is possible that a few abnormal cells may have been present at birth and it takes many years of cell division and reproduction to produce a significant mass of cells sufficient to be recognizable as a tumour; but the nucleus of the original ovum is not recognizable as cancerous. It simply carries the defect which switches on the nuclear change in certain cells at a later stage of development.

More evidence is coming to light from studies of the blood groups of patients with certain types of cancer indicating a genetic disposition to cancer. As part of the defence mechanism of the body, which will be considered later, the fluid part of the blood, the plasma, contains chemicals which destroy red cells from other species or other humans when they are introduced into the blood stream. Not from all humans; for some individuals are compatible in this respect, one with another; others are not. This is why blood has to be tested or 'grouped' before a blood transfusion is given. Every individual has his special genetic imprint displayed by his blood groups which are part of his individuality inherited from his father and mother. Some cancers have been shown to be more commonly associated with certain blood groups thus indicating, at least, that genetic factors affected their development.

Familial cancer is not common and we must presume that most cancer is acquired in the rough and tumble of our environment. It will be rougher, for instance, in space; it is rougher on earth after atmospheric pollution from nuclear (in the physical not the biological sense) bombardment of Hiroshima, Nagasaki and all those tests. At all times from birth – and sometimes before if a mother is X-rayed injudiciously during pregnancy – our cell nuclei are at risk of change and mutilation.

One of the microscopic manifestations in the nucleus of malignant change is an increase in the number of chromosomes. Polyploidy is a change well known to horticulturists who obtain bigger and better specimens by doubling or trebling the number of chromosomes in plants. The polyploid cell in man would contain a multiple of 46 chromosomes but in cancer the excess is more variable – aneuploidy. In man 'normal' tissue examined under the microscope will show a small proportion of random aneuploid cells at all times. These mostly come to nothing; but a high proportion of the cells of a tumour are aneuploid and the nuclear material of the rest of its cells looks distorted, even swollen and abnormal. Throughout life cells are being bent towards cancer as a result of the hazards of our environment and are presenting in cancerous form. Many do not survive nor reproduce themselves but as time passes the quantum of abnormal cells can increase beyond control.

The secret of cancer, if there is one, lies in the nucleus. The clues of its origin have already been given. The mature red cell does not become cancerous – because it has no nucleus. By inference cancer is therefore a disease arising from the cell nucleus. But this is not enough. The only other tissues in the body from which cancer does not grow are the nerves and the heart. Cancers do occur from the tissues which support the nerve cell and surround it – the insulation, as it were – but never from the nerve itself. Nor from the muscle of the heart. These are the only tissues in the body in which the cells are permanent, which do not require to be replaced during life. The nuclei of their cells maintain function but do not need to replicate. Therefore they do not need to divide. From which we may conclude that cancerous change takes place in nuclei at an un-guarded moment–when the nuclei divide. At that moment they are vulnerable to improper change from external influences – external to their cells though not always external to the body itself.

CHAPTER THREE

Associated Factors in Cancer

It is hardly possible to distinguish 'normal' in human biological affairs and the concept that we are born into life normal and may by ill-chance transgress and step over the border into abnormal is a simplism which is no longer tenable. In medicine, however, we do have to make this distinction which is usually clear and only sometimes blurred and uncertain; though as we delve deeper and find out more so we become less certain. We talk of abnormality being pathological – an abnormal cell is usually pathological, a cancer cell is certainly pathological. It can be seen to be abnormal under the microscope since it differs recognizably from the usual appearance. We talk of a pathological situation when a system or a series of systems goes out of order. Under such circumstances it may be possible to see pathological change in the cells of the organs concerned, sometimes it may not. Conversely abnormal cells may be seen which are not apparently causing any ill effect; it may then be difficult to regard this as a pathological state despite the evidence of the microscope. A case in point is ageing. It is inevitable to grow old and so, presumably, normal to do so. Yet ageing, in cellular terms, appears to be pathological.

Ageing is a complex process which is displayed in several ways. The most obvious effect is in the arteries. Relatively early in life, long before the individual could be considered to be getting old, let alone middle aged, a pathological change begins in the wall of the larger arteries. Abnormal material is deposited, patchily at first, more generally later, in and under the smooth lining of these tubes. The vessels lose their elasticity and gradually silt up. Sometimes the silting is abrupt leading to a coronary thrombosis when an artery in the heart is blocked, a stroke when one to the brain is obstructed. But there are less disastrous effects.

The blood contained within the arteries serves numerous functions of supply which are vital to the individual cells. It brings fuel and oxygen so that the fuel can be burnt to supply energy, to enable the cell to survive and to work. In the case of secretory cells it carries the raw materials with which the cell can fabricate its product. It also carries special chemicals which activate function, the chemical messengers known as hormones.

Gradual deprivation of blood supply results in failure of tissues to replace themselves adequately. In muscle the mass of its component cell fibres can no longer be sustained by the diminishing supply and wasting occurs. That simply means fewer cells, but in muscle the cells, seen individually, change little if at all as regards their nuclei. It is probably no coincidence that muscle cancer is very rare, and then as often as not is due to an inherited genetic disorder.

But not so elsewhere. Some tissues show as a phenomenon of ageing a high incidence of cells with abnormality within their nuclei. This is very unlikely to be due to the deprivation of blood; the nuclear change is just part of ageing, and the tissues most affected by this phenomenon are also those most prone to cancer. Moreover, the nuclear abnormalities seen in increasing number as years go by are very like those which distinguish cancer cells, and though the forms in which these abnormalities present themselves are varied, no single variety is to be seen in preference to any other in either ageing or cancer.

This is not to say that the one always begets the other

for though the nuclear changes are always there with age cancer does not always occur. Maybe ageing sets the stage on which malignancy can more readily develop. Much circumstantial evidence links the two. If mice are submitted to the effects of X-rays their cells show the usual stigmata of ageing. Human beings have sometimes inadvertently received more X-rays than is good for them when they are young – in the uterus when the mother is being investigated or even as misplaced treatment of some innocent condition. Subsequent investigation has revealed that malignancy occurs at an abnormally high incidence at an early age and at unusual sites.

At sites where cancer is common its incidence is notably higher as age proceeds; for example in England and Wales the incidence of skin cancer is approximately 50 per 100,000 at the age of 50 but has risen to 200 per 100,000 at 70. But there are exceptions and this – the fact and its exception – present an explanation.

The nuclear deformities of age may either be due to the development of senescence or may represent the cellular scars of disease encountered and overcome – that rough and tumble which ensues from the competition between all living things with one another, between animal kingdom, bacteria and viruses, and with their chemical and physical environment. Our environment can push cells the whole way through to cancer; or it may initiate new generations of abnormal cell-lines without the power to invade but susceptible to later attack by another agent. A virus may set the premalignant course, so that generations of cells can be maintained in a premalignant state for years without further change; then exposure to further nuclear damage gives the cell another push towards malignancy. Fully developed cancer cells are born.

But there are cancers, common ones in fact, which develop with increasing frequency for a time and then at a certain age their rising incidence is checked and may even fall in some types. Breast cancer is a good example. The overall incidence of this growth increases as age proceeds but the *rate* of increase changes. The rate is steep to the age of 40 and just over; thereafter the rate of increase is reduced to almost half. Two factors must be at work. There is the ageing process dominant throughout the life span. The added factor enhancing the rate to the age of 40 comes, surprisingly perhaps, from within the individual.

The steeply rising incidence coincides with the active reproductive period in women (breast cancer is hardly seen in the vestigial breast tissue possessed by men). It is not unreasonable to think therefore that it may in some way be connected with those chemical substances produced by certain sex glands to regulate the rhythmic changes of the menstrual cycle and pregnancy. These are the sex hormones. A hormone is simply a chemical substance created within special cells, which initiates activity in other cells; and a hormone reaches its target from its source by way of the blood stream. A hormone is, in fact, a chemical messenger. For example, oestrogens are a group of hormones developed in the ovary which take part with others in regulating changes in the uterus associated with the menstrual cycle. These and other sex hormones dominate the scene between puberty and menopause, and in this period their activity, particularly the oestrogens, boosts the number of breast cancer cases. This is why it is sometimes necessary to remove the ovaries in the treatment of breast cancer – and even go further by giving male sex hormones, the androgens, to neutralize, as it were, any oestrogenic effect from other glands after the ovaries have been removed – for the ovaries are not the sole source of supply.

So here is a new factor in the genesis of cancer – an intrinsic factor. We create within ourselves chemical substances which dispose some of our own tissues to cancer. In the ethos of the perfection of the human body which regards health and disease as two opposing poles, as states of grace and disgrace, this idea must appear outrageous, almost cannibalistic. It is, however, yet another example that the concept of normal and abnormal provides only a rough working philosophy on which we may construct the pathological basis of medicine; and another instance that cancer is no affliction from outside but an inevitable consequence of biological life.

There are other hormonal influences in the genesis of breast cancer. Back in the early eighteenth century a keen observer noted breast cancer to be commoner in nuns. Rather more than two centuries later an international study has reaffirmed this and demonstrated considerable variation in incidence between one country and another. Seven centres were involved in an investigation covering the U.S.A., Formosa, Japan, Greece, Brazil, Yugoslavia and Wales. In the U.S.A. the incidence is twenty-six cases each year per 100,000 women, in Japan and Formosa as low as four. It proves better to be married than single, better still to have a baby and best of all to have it early. The risks in the single woman are a third higher than those who are married; on probing deeper this appears to be related to child-bearing. A surprising fact is the relationship between the age at which a woman has her first child and the possibility of her developing cancer of the breast. The risk in a woman starting her family at the age of 18 is one-third what it would be if she started when 35. It may be that pregnancy early in life changes the pattern of that group of hormones referred to earlier, the oestrogens, in a way that favours the harmless ones at the expense of those which do the damage.

Then there is the milk factor first discovered two decades or so ago in mice. It was found that the offspring of a strain of mice prone to breast cancer developed the disease if they were breast-fed but not if they were separated from their mothers at the moment of birth. Furthermore the cancers developed not immediately but later in life – at the usual time in fact. So there was a transmissible factor in the milk either lying dormant in the body of the offspring for years or starting the nuclear change in infancy which then progressed slowly to become manifest later – a possibility which will be discussed later (Chapter Ten). Now reports from the U.S.A. and India point to a similar situation in humans and indict as the culprit a special virus, named the Bittner virus, which has been found commonly in women with a family history of cancer and uncommonly in those without. In Bombay there is an inbred Persian population known as the Parsi. Breast cancer is much more common in Parsi women than in the indigenous Indian population and the Bittner virus has been found in as many as 40 per cent of Parsi women.

The breast is not the only tissue which exhibits the phenomenon of an internal cause for cancer. Cancer of the uterine cervix develops with increasing incidence, again until the age of about 40. Thereafter it does not behave quite like the breast, for after 40 the incidence does not increase at all. This is not to say that cancer of the cervix does not occur thereafter; it continues to develop in the population at the same rate – the incidence levels off. It would appear that a hormonal influence is switched off at the menopause, nevertheless leaving some individuals whose cells were affected when the hormone was active but in whom the resulting cancerous development was slower. The cancer becomes manifest in them only as the years roll by.

All this seems to put women at a considerable disadvantage; but men are not exempt from hormone-dependent cancers. There is the prostate where cancer is

23

encouraged by the male hormones, the androgens. So the situation is complementary to cancer of the breast in women though, in contrast to breast cancer, the incidence of prostatic cancer increases with age with no slackening off at the age of 40 – perhaps because men have no sudden menopause. To treat prostatic cancer the androgens can either be reduced by removal of the testicles or by neutralization with oestrogens. For obvious reasons the latter is the treatment of choice.

The testis behaves differently; unlike breast, uterus or prostate, it is a site uncommon for cancer. But when this does occur it virtually starts from puberty and increases in incidence at the same steep rate until the fourth decade of life when the incidence falls back equally steeply until at 70 it almost reaches the prepubertal base. If we can suppose a male climacteric, a gradual andropause, and if testicular cancer is hormone induced, why should it not imitate the uterine cervical pattern? Probably because it is ordained, not by ageing, but by the antithesis, growth, for cell turnover is necessarily greater in developing tissue. Though the rising incidence of testicular cancer starts at puberty, it relents at an age too early to be regarded as the male climacteric. It looks, therefore, as though cancer may develop here from the conjunction of hormonal activity upon cells in a highly active state of development, when they are rapidly reproducing themselves. The effect is seen immediately in the rate of increase; this continues into the two decades of life following puberty because of individual variability in the time required for the cancer to become manifest.

The vulnerability of normal tissue cells in growth is also a feature of bone, and here growth alone seems to be the principal factor. Again, bone is a rare site for the disease, rarer in fact than the testis. But teenage life presents a peak incidence, albeit only 2 per 100,000 males each year, com-

24

pared with 6 per 100,000 for the testis at the peak of its incidence at 35 years. By 20 years of age the incidence for bone is falling and it is not until 50 that the disease recurs significantly. Clearly bone in later life is subject to the influences already discussed which complicate, confuse and distort cell replication as the years pass. But at the beginning of life the situation can only be explained by development, not ageing, by the demand for cell multiplication and the strains placed upon the cell nucleus dividing with such greater frequency. For the bones at this age must grow and it is especially significant that it is what are known as the long bones which are affected then. The long bones support our limbs, they are the bones which add to our stature and, in the lower limbs particularly, most rapidly develop their girth to support the weight of the erect being. At about 20-years-old their growing cartilaginous caps begin to fuse into bone and disappear so that growth ceases; at the same time the incidence of cancer ceases to rise, falls back and within a few years is at less than 1 per 100,000.

But these are uncommon sites for cancer, worthy of attention only as regards the light they shed upon its cause, or rather its development, since in biological affairs there is no such finality as cause. The search for cause leads only to infinity; as soon as a cause is found a reason must be sought for the mechanisms behind that cause.

Cancer of the breast is in the common group. Unseen before puberty it starts in the third decade and develops in over 100 per 100,000 women at age 45, and just less than 200 at 80. Cancer of the lung is worse, beginning to rise in the fourth decade of life and contributing over 400 per 100,000 persons at the seventh decade (both sexes are affected but men more than women). The lung has given more evidence of causative factors of cancer than other sites. That cigarette smoking is the *deus ex machina* is now common knowledge. The evidence of a direct correlation between cancer and both the duration of smoking and the quantity smoked is conclusive. The earlier in life the habit is formed, the longer it is maintained and the heavier the smoking, the greater the chance of malignant change. If the habit is broken the malignant spell is broken, almost but not quite – the incidence in those who break the habit ceases to rise.

Cigarette smoking is the best known of the causes of cancer, established as a fact by clinical study. There is other information. The prevalence of lung cancer is recent; it has grown in concert with the habit. By the late nineteenth and early twentieth centuries both habit and the growth were uncommon and particularly so in women. The occurrence of lung cancer in women is more recent than in men and tallies with the change in social mores which has permitted women to take to the cigarette.

Cancers at other sites have also demonstrated rise and decline indicative of changes possibly in social habit or environment which have introduced agents of nuclear damage we are unaware of, or withdrawn them from under our very noses leaving us innocent of their nature, whence they came or where they went. The next ten to twenty years will possibly see a change in the incidence of cancer of the cervix uteri – a change for the worse, for there is increasing evidence both in women and the mouse that the 'pill', which is a hormone, may have a cancerous effect both here and perhaps on the breast. A balance may be brought about at the uterine site by our increasing ability with the aid of samples taken at well-women clinics to detect the change which precedes frank malignancy and deal with it before it has bolted into malignancy – but more of this anon (Chapter Eight).

For many years the association between cancer and chemicals has been obvious. The soot clinging to the

26

creases of the scrotal skin of sweeps in the days when they climbed chimneys led to scrotal cancer as does the oil which soaks the clothes of men in heavy industry – first seen in the operatives of mules in the cotton industry. A substance known as α-naphthylamine used in rubber manufacture promotes cancer in the bladder. Even the drug, L.S.D., used by addicts for kicks, alters cell nuclei in a way that may promote cancer. Betel, which many chew incessantly in India and beyond gives rise to cancer in the mouth. Betel, as chewed, is a conjunction of tobacco and lime rolled up in the betel leaf. If this can have direct effect upon the mouth, may there not be other cancerous agents in what we eat?

The harmful agents in soot and oil are certain hydrocarbons; oils and fats used in frying could be converted by the heat to similar substances but of this there is no proof, despite some desultory research. In fact little evidence has been sought in this field where the increasing use of preservatives are giving cause for concern – as the cyclamates, to give one example.

Fourteen years ago nitrosamines, formed as a compound from nitrites and certain amines, were shown to cause liver tumours in mice. Moreover, there was more than a hint that one dose was sufficient to start the cancerous ball rolling. Nitrates are an inevitable part of our diet and these can become converted to nitrites in food preservation. And nitrates are used as meat preservatives. On the other side the significant amines are formed in alcoholic fermentation, tobacco smoke and fish products. The two, the nitrites and the amines, can combine in gastric juice; so we may from time to time unwittingly ingest this cancerogenic substance.

A deficiency of molybdenum in the soil where nitrates are used as fertilizers leads to nitrite accumulation in plants and vegetables. Molybdenum deficiency is present

27

in Transkei, in South Africa; cancer of the gullet is notable there and nitrosamines have been detected in food plants of the area. Before 1950 this cancer was seldom seen in the Bantu; 20 per cent of hospital admissions affecting Bantus are now registered for treatment of oesophageal (gullet) cancer. And to round the story off, one particular nitrosamine compound causes oesophageal cancer in rats whether given by mouth or by injection .

Sometimes the cancerous agent is created for us by the action of fungi. It is not long since aflotoxin, a substance created by the mould *Aspergillus flavus*, was shown to be responsible for the development of liver tumours in trout. It also accounted for an epidemic of liver disease but not cancers in turkeys leading to the death of 100,000 birds in 1960–61 due to deterioration of food-stuffs by this mould. It is not inconceivable that contamination with *Aspergillus* and so aflotoxin does from time to time affect cereals kept in store for human consumption.

Cancer of the gullet and stomach are commonly seen in the East, a fact ascribed more by hypothesis than proof to repeated ingestion of overhot food, or to spices. There is also good reason to believe that repeated injury to the gullet occurs in other ways seen more in the East than the West. Observe how a chicken is prepared for the table in Hong Kong. It is cut up regardless of the bone structure, with the result that numerous small splinters of bone are inadvertently swallowed and these lead to repeated abrasion sometimes even to perforation of the lower part of the gullet. The custom is not confined to Hong Kong or the hen.

In the 1930s gastric cancer was twice as common in Holland and the U.S.A. than in England, the English interpretation of this being the greater prevalence of spirit drinking in those countries. This interpretation was probably prejudice. The incidence of cancer at any site you can

28

think of tends to vary from country to country. For example large bowel cancer, which it would be difficult to attribute to alcohol since this is absorbed before the intestinal contents reach the large intestine, develops in 45 persons per 100,000 in U.S.A., 31 in Canada, 24 in England, 8 in Japan and 6 in Nigeria. However, these figures do correlate with living standards. A higher fat content in the food carries bile and its salts, which are discharged into the small intestine and usually broken down there, further down into the large intestine with the result that the bacterial content in the colon changes. There are reasons to suppose that a particular group of bacteria, known as bacteroides, may dispose to cancer and this group can colonize the large intestine in the presence of bile salts.

Spirits, too, have been blamed for cancer which starts in the liver, hardly seen here but common in the U.S.A. Alcoholism leads to cirrhosis and wherever cirrhosis of the liver is common liver cancer tends to develop, the simple view being that either the inflammation or the scar tissue in the liver can develop into malignancy, just as it can in the bladder of patients with bilharzia due to infestation with a parasite from the waters of the Nile. For cancer sometimes occurs in longstanding inflammation and old scars elsewhere, on the skin for example.

And the skin is susceptible just to the effects of sunlight and particularly ultra-violet light. Skin cancer is more often seen in outdoor workers, particularly of fair complexion; moreover, it develops in exposed areas unprotected by clothing. The incidence is high in Australia particularly so in sunbathers so that attempts have been made to discourage this practice. Melanoma, a skin cancer rare here, which incorporates the pigment cell, is also common in Australia; and this in a population for the most part genetically the same as in these isles. Moreover, its incidence increases from south to north as the light intensity increases towards the equator.

Scar tissue itself is, however, unlikely to provide the cells from which a cancer grows, for where scars and cancer occur together the cellular elements of the tumour are clearly derived from the tissue of origin, be it liver or skin, and do not resemble the reparative scar cells. The large intestine is subject to a chronic inflammatory disease, ulcerative colitis; the risk of cancer of the large intestine is thirty times higher for those who have had this disease for ten years or more than for those of a similar age-group who have had no such trouble. The growth clearly originates from the epithelial cell which lines the bowel, not from scar tissue. The explanation probably lies in the high turnover of epithelial cells needed to repair the ulceration. A quicker turnover would provide greater opportunity for new generations of cells to arise and so for cells with abnormal nuclei. In this disease before a growth develops cells can be found, not frankly malignant but distinctly odd, which to the experienced eye are pre-malignant.

It is peculiar therefore that cancer is so rare in the small intestine for here there is a naturally rapid turnover of epithelium, the most rapid anywhere in the body. Even when the small intestinal mucosa is diseased and inflamed, as it is sometimes, it does not become malignant. By contrast cancer does arise in the stomach and is more inclined to do so when its lining has been abnormal for some time and has reached the degenerate state of atrophy. The explanation may lie in the fact that intestinal epithelial cells are constantly shed into the lumen of the gut; an aberrant cell would therefore be lost before it could reproduce itself and gain a foothold.

So cancer is not a single entity for which a single cause can be found. Like infection, it covers a whole range of disease, is a disordered response, mostly to environment in the widest sense and has many causes. Some tissues are more susceptible than others and this susceptibility has a close relationship to the source of origin of those tissues as they developed from ovum to embryo.

Mention was made in Chapter Two of how the original totipotential cell divided to make two cells, then four and so on. Almost imperceptibly this little knot of cells begins to show that it is organized and there appear three main groups of cells, each with its different structure and ultimate function within the body. The cells which ensheath the little solid ball all appropriately provide the coat or lining of the full-grown body. Those which are turned in when invagination of the mass occurs are the endoderm; from these develop the epithelial cells which line the gut from mouth to anus. Those which remain on the outside, now the ectoderm, provide the epithelium of the skin. Cancer is much more common in tissues which have their origin in ectoderm and endoderm. This may at first seem odd since so many cancers are internal – in the breast, the prostate and the gut. But those cells which provide the secretion of glands such as the breast or the innumerable glands in the mucous membranes of the alimentary system are derived, by invaginations late in development, from ecto- or endoderm.

The mesoderm, that is the cells forming the internal mass of the very early embryo, is the origin of the cells of all supporting structures – muscles, bones, arteries, blood cells; and that filler material which holds organs together in their general shape, known as fibrous tissue. Cancer from mesoderm – sarcoma – is rare; cancer of blood vessels is almost never seen. Oddly, when mesothelium becomes cancerous it does so at an earlier age than epithelium and the cancer is in general more virulent. This may be a consequence of blood supply of those parts rather than a reflection of embryonic origin; this effect of blood supply on the virulence will be considered in Chapter Four.

Leukaemia, which affects the white cells and is therefore a cancer of mesoderm, is a more common disease than sarcoma. Perhaps this is because the normal white cell exists for a shorter time than other normal mesodermal cells before being replaced. Consequently the cell turnover of white cells is more rapid presenting a greater opportunity for abnormal nuclear change. This change tends to affect the parent cells from which the white cells are developed and matured before being used in the circulating blood. The disease develops at any age throughout life affecting babies (Chapter Ten) and the elderly. The disease in old age is a cancer of the mature white cell in the blood, the lymphocyte. Notwithstanding the cancerous appearances of these leukaemic cells the disease is hardly malignant in its effects – in contrast to other forms of leukaemia occurring earlier in life.

While the white cells have nuclei, the red cell, as it circulates in the blood, has not. So there is no cancer of the mature red cell. However, new red cells have constantly to be provided from babyhood until death and this is achieved from nucleated parent cells which are found mostly within the bone marrow. These can go wrong in an almost malignant manner and so produce an uncommon disease in which too many red cells are delivered to and circulate in the blood.

These facts only serve to emphasize that cancer is a disease of the cell nucleus. The evidence of nuclear aberration is all too clear in myeloid leukaemia. Here abnormality of one of the pairs of chromosomes can actually be seen. Further confirmation that this chromosomal abnormality is responsible comes from study of mongoloid children.

The chief chromosomal abnormality in mongols, and indeed the cause of the condition, is an extra chromosome. An error occurs in that stage of cell division which creates single instead of paired chromosomes in order to provide ova or spermatozoa. All pairs should divide and separate at this stage, but by chance one of the smaller pairs fails to separate so that the resulting gamete (ovum or spermatozoa) has 24 instead of 23 chromosomes and on meeting its opposite gamete at fertilization a final cell of 47 chromosomes is formed, with three chromosomes in one pair where only two should be. This abnormal chromosomal 'pair' which gives rise to mongolism is the same as the one sometimes seen to be deformed but not over-number in one form of leukaemia. It will come as no surprise, therefore, that the incidence of leukaemia is high in mongoloid children.

This is not to say that every case of leukaemia has this abnormality as its cause. Indeed, recent research has revealed viruses to be involved. The nuclear protein of certain viruses can take over the D.N.A. (Chapter Two) of the white cell and so become part of the genetic apparatus of that cell converting it into a leukaemic cell.

The white cell is also particularly susceptible to irradiation; leukaemia can result from overdosage due to X-ray investigation, X-ray treatment or fall-out after atomic explosions. Space travel has this as an added worry since the earth's atmosphere ordinarily shields us from most of the baneful effects of solar radiation.

So cancer is as natural to us as living because it arises out of growth, ageing, even the chemical hormonal systems within us – and because of our environment.

CHAPTER FOUR

Spread of Cancer

There are benign growths and malignant ones. A benign growth, even though it often presents as a tumour, cannot really be regarded as cancer. For cancer is a very general term to indicate an invasive disease in which the growth by one means or another invades the normal tissues of the host. A wart is an example of a benign growth, and though it is a matter of common observation that warts on the fingers, for example, grow larger and even produce little seedlings near by, so that they seem to spread, they do not invade and destroy the individual. In fact they represent the reaction of that outer part of the skin known as the epidermis to a virus which has implanted itself in the skin.

So perhaps a wart is not a good example of a benign growth for really it represents an infection and not an apparently spontaneous new growth, although warts in the bladder are disposed to become malignant. One of the commonest benign tumours lies under the skin in the fat and is an agglomeration of fat cells forming a lipoma. We do not know why this happens, any more than why the secretory cells of the female breast may also sometimes develop simple, that is benign, tumours. But we do know that they do not spread but stay where they are with no evidence of any desire to trespass beyond a capsule which usually encloses them. And the only thing to be said against them is that they may tend to get bigger in the course of time, simply because the cells inside them, which resemble in every way those of the normal tissue they arise from, continue to reproduce themselves without stopping.

But in the wide variety of cancers, some are more malignant than others – a simple statement requiring expansion since it conceals the whole philosophy of malignancy; and this is not easy to define. Malignancy reflects the power of uncontrolled multiplication of the cells of a tumour at the expense of the host. But it must be more than this, since such a lesion could provide a localized tumour confined to its original site – a mere wen, an irritating bump. Invasiveness provides the basis of malignant quality. Yet we do not regard bacterial invasion as malignant and bacteria can reduplicate and invade very much at the expense of the host. Bacteria can spread from the original site of infection directly through tissue and along the vascular channels of communication; so can malignant cells. The means of attack are the same even to the fact that both bacteria and malignant cells may develop chemicals deleterious to the host or utilize his metabolic processes to their gain and his loss. Both are therefore 'malignant'; but the cancer cell has arisen from within the individual himself. The bacterium or virus is a living organism in its own right, a separate entity which exists by invading us and clearly has some existence outside the body. But in cancer the malignant cell arises from within us from normal cells going wrong when they reproduce themselves. The cause of this may lie outside the body, though not always, but the invader is a rogue cell – from our own tissues that have been caused to turn upon us.

Like bacterial invasion the virulence of cancer is infinitely variable. The boil is a nuisance; it seldom gets out of hand, but is contained locally. Similarly the rodent ulcer, a common form of skin cancer also stays put. Yet it is malignant for its cells, epithelial cells, can be seen to be out of place lying in little nests beneath the surface; but the invasion stops there. A look at those cells shows them to be very like their parent tissue, the nuclei much the same, the cytoplasm little different, even the shape of the cells little changed. These malignant cells have almost developed to what their normal counterparts look like under the microscope. As already observed the cells of each tissue look different, their shape usually reflecting their function. This differentiation is well maintained in less malignant growths – in fact we speak of well-differentiated growths. And here is an important feature of the range of malignancy. The more malignant, the more invasive the lesion, the more undifferentiated the cell; that is the less like its normal ancestor it has become. Its nucleus is irregular, large and active; it travels light as regards cytoplasm; its shape is variable and hardly recognizable as what it should have been; at its most malignant it is economically round. With this lack of differentiation the cell bears no resemblance to the tissue the cancer is developing in.

Whether it be the gut or the breast, the range of differentiation varies from one cancer to another. Although there is a general tendency to good differentiation in the skin for example – and skin cancers are amongst the less malignant – in the stomach it is often otherwise; they are usually poorly differentiated and more malignant. Age also has a part in this for cancers developing at a younger age tend to be less well differentiated. So one growth may display the quietism and near control of its parent tissue, another shows the vigorous development, the cell activity, even the anonymity which paradoxically gives the undifferentiated growth its character.

Malignancy is not simply a matter of the ability of the cancerous cells to invade the body generally, to spread through its transport systems to set up new secondary growths (known as metastases) elsewhere. The power of

36

the cells of the tumour, or its satellites elsewhere, to push out into the tissue in which it lies at the expense of the normal surrounding cells is the fundamental element of malignancy. And this is curious; or perhaps more curious is the self-control in this respect shown by normal cells.

In most tissues (Chapter Two) the component cells replace themselves and have the power to do so to make good loss either by damage or by simple cell decline and death, for in many tissues cell life is finite and much shorter than the span of the whole man. Why then if cells of the liver, say, go on reproducing themselves do they ever stop? Why do they not just go on and on so that the liver gets bigger and bigger? We do not know; but there seems to be a controlling mechanism in the cells which switches off when the organ concerned is fully developed and equipped, and switches on when more tissue is needed. This control appears to be exercised in the form of an inhibition. When the cells have fitted the space they should occupy their juxtaposition to one another, or perhaps the pressure or tension they create within the organ, does the trick. There is no proof of this; it provides a convenient supposition for understanding. The process is called contact inhibition, the idea being that it is the contact of one normal cell against another which holds them in check.

So normal cells create their own self-limitation both in normal tissue and benign tumours; not so malignant cells. Contact inhibition is lost in cancer. Malignant cells go on reproducing, not necessarily at any faster rate than normal cells but quite unchecked. Two things result. The malignant cells push out in between their normal companions and they fail to fall together in the architectural pattern particular to the organ concerned, for if contact inhibition is lost the cells cannot be arranged in the usual manner.

The rate at which the malignant cell replicates is unknown. It has always been assumed that it outpaces the normal cell but evidence is beginning to accumulate that this is not so in some cancers. Perhaps there is variability in this too; in some cancers the cells go ahead faster than the normal cells of the tissue or organ involved, in others not. However, the degree of malignancy, that is the invasiveness, of a growth goes hand in hand with the poorness of differentiation of its cells and it is possible that there are degrees of contact inhibition, which may be partially lost in the less malignant, better differentiated growth and completely so in the most malignant, most undifferentiated lesions. And to some extent the more malignant growths defeat themselves for they outreach the supply of blood they need so that the cells in the centre are starved of oxygen and nutrients with the result that they die leaving the centre of the tumour necrotic.

Spread is first local into the interstices of the tissue and organ which harbour it. About the methods of spread beyond the original tumour there is no mystery; the transport systems are there for normal function and these are used by cancer cells. Perhaps the mystery lies in the obverse – why do not normal cells break off from their proper position, circulate and prosper round the corner? They do trespass sometimes when forced out by injury – muscle cells in particular and globules of fat. But they do not implant and grow. Fat can damage by blocking small capillary vessels. Muscle cells cause little trouble partly because the little fragment of tissue is often too large to gain access to the small vessels, but also because normal cells do not implant themselves elsewhere where they would be out of context. (Grafting is different since the tissue is placed where it should be; whole organ transplant is another matter.) This is where the malignant cell has the edge; it can implant, is capable of independent growth and can take possession.

All tissues are provided with a dual service of supply.

Every need for cellular activity is carried in the first; through the arteries, then the smaller capillaries, the accessory materials flow to where the cells are lodged and bathed in fluid. The cellular components of the blood remain in the vascular channels except the white cells of the smaller variety which move out if needed into the fluid around the tissue cells. There would be no purpose in the red cells leaving the blood vessels since their sole function is to provide oxygen which can diffuse through the vessel wall and tissue fluid to the cells of the tissue itself. The smaller white cells, the lymphocytes, have another purpose which will be considered later (Chapter Seven). While oxygen and the materials for the proper function of the cells are carried thus in solution across to the tissue, chemicals and fluid the cells have discarded go back by the same route to the capillaries and so are decanted into the veins where they meet the red cells again, after these have lost their oxygen. The larger white cells are retained under ordinary circumstances within the blood vessels though when they are needed it is beside the tissue cell itself and then they must pass out of the vessels. Normally all blood vessel walls are safely guarded to prevent leakage of red cells; the larger white cells therefore have to be released by the process of inflammation which causes a breach by damaging the capillary wall. Inevitably where infection develops and these white cells are needed red cells leak out also. Only rarely does a cancer incite inflammation, usually a sign of a virulent growth, though inflammation does occur when bacterial infection complicates a growth.

The lymphatic system provides the second means of drainage. Lymphatics, the main ones, are small tubes, not as small as capillaries which can only be seen under the microscope, but infinitely smaller than the arteries and vessels alongside which they lie. Lymph nodes interrupt at intervals as filter beds and more; at these nodes, or glands as they are commonly called, the lymphocyte cell develops, a cell of prime importance in defence and immunity which acts not only in the nodes but throughout the body. The lymphocyte is carried within the blood stream and also in the lymphatic fluid, which flows on through node after node and eventually pours by one main duct back into a main vein near the heart. It would be a mistake to regard it as a subsidiary venous return, not just because it carries no red cells, but because the system has a purpose other than transport, namely defence. It picks up bacteria and consumes them; it provides the immunological cell with its vast potential of adaptation needed to mitigate the effects of entry of foreign protein into the body, whether in bacterial or other form, and to render impotent the cancer cell. The cancer cell is not, as the emotive fear would have us think, inviolable; many such cells which wander into the blood stream or through the lymphatics disappear.

Malignancy is disorder and follows the laws of disorder. Its spread is therefore not entirely predictable for many factors are involved some of which we can understand, others not. Clearly the vigour and power of the cell to reproduce – the supply of cells, in fact – ordains both local invasiveness and the power to spread beyond, while accessibility of the blood stream must further enhance the possibility of dissemination. Cells in any tissue are fed through tissue fluid which flows slowly to lymphatics. Within this fluid cancer cells can float away along the lymphatic route and spread to the nearest chain of lymph nodes in an orderly way. Cancer of the skin can be seen to be orderly in its invasion because these growths are not at the outset close to blood vessels of adequate calibre; and they filter slowly and predictably along the lymphatic system.

An exception in the skin is the rodent ulcer, an unfortunate name derived from earlier days when treatment was often long delayed. These growths spread neither by blood stream nor by lymphatics probably because they gain access to neither. So they are capable only of slow local invasiveness and are limited to ulceration commonly seen on the face or scalp. If allowed to persist for a considerable time, ulceration deepens eroding through the skin and beyond – hence 'rodent' ulcer with its macabre implication, as much an insult to man as to the rat. The name is doubly unfortunate since it reinforces the emotive sense of cancer in a growth that is particularly benign and few ulcers of this type progress thus far today. Many basal-cell lesions, the pathological category in which the rodent ulcer falls, live quietly and innocuously with their host; moreover, the lesion is common, sufficiently common to be observed by a sharp eye on any ordinary day's peregrinations. A common cancer and no cause for fear; the cells are well differentiated and stay out of harm's way. More serious is the melanoma, a skin cancer which is pigmented. It is rare in England, but in Australia is common and recent study there has shown it to behave predictably and its spread to be lymphatically ordained in the earlier part of its existence.

Elsewhere disorder and so unpredictability is more in evidence. This is a matter of blood supply, for an organ richly bathed in blood is likely, if it harbours cancer, to shed malignant cells into the blood stream. General dissemination then occurs. The stomach is an example. It is rich in both blood and lymph; its function demands this on account of its considerable volume of secretion, which can only come from the blood, and its considerable absorption. Though a wide range of cellular differentiation is displayed here the odds are very much against containment of the growth. It cannot but spread via the blood to liver and beyond, via lymphatic channels to the main duct and so again into the main veins. And so gastric cancer spreads more rapidly with greater disorder because of wider dissemination of its cells.

By contrast, at the other end of the gut progress is slow for the mucosa of the rectum is concerned only with secretion of mucus and is not involved in the considerable turnover necessary for digestion. There is some absorption but it is not great – a little fluid and a little salt. The natural history of rectal cancer is very much longer and the outcome better than stomach cancer. A man may outlive his rectal cancer, another end may well take him. Not so for stomach.

The effect of blood supply is further demonstrated in organs where its flow varies from time to time. Sometimes a cancer develops during pregnancy or was present unsuspected when pregnancy began. During pregnancy and lactation which follows it, the blood supply of the breast increases vastly to meet the obvious functional need of secreting milk. A cancer arising in the midst of this is bad not so much due to an increasing virulence of the cells but because the cells being richly supplied can multiply easily and can all too quickly reach the blood stream and disseminate far and wide.

Containment is also a matter of anatomy and propinquity, of whether the affected organ lies cheek by jowl with other susceptible tissues; for some tissues are less susceptible to penetration, or seem so. Take the gut for example. It is suspended in coils within the abdomen. The cavity which contains the intestine is lined throughout with a thin, shining, smooth coat, a membrane in fact to reduce friction to a minimum. This, the peritoneum, also covers the coils of intestine, or most of it, and enables one part to glide over the next without difficulty. Thus the peritoneum tends to isolate one coil from another and prevent a growth spreading directly from one loop to the

42

next. A growth in the bowel will for much of its existence remain within its original site spreading by its blood and lymph channels but not to what lies adjacent, though as it becomes advanced and eventually breaks through, cells float into the peritoneal cavity where some may implant on other organs.

A growth at the edge of the lung can be held for a time by the pleura on its surface, another membrane just like peritoneum with the same purpose. It spreads more easily through the lung tissue and its root, which is not covered by pleura. But the gullet passes through the centre of the chest between the lungs and has no pleural cover. There it lies in close proximity to neighbouring structures, sharing blood and lymph supply with them. Transgression from the primary site all too easily occurs. Likewise the pancreas, essentially a part of the alimentary system despite its insulin role, is a thin solid organ plastered on to the structures which form the back wall of the abdomen behind the peritoneum. There is little to stop direct spread of the primary growth there and it seldom does even though years may have elapsed from its onset (their duration is difficult to judge since these cancers are, like others, frequently painless and only make their presence felt at a late stage). This is why cancers in the gullet and the pancreas are difficult to excise and survivors are few.

Tissue tension, that is the actual pressure which cells themselves exert upon one another and what surrounds them is another matter. As a growth develops with multiplication of cells competition for space occurs, tissue tension rises. Thus the passage of its cells as they erode into a blood vessel is assisted, *vis à tergo*, by a purely physical effect. Place the growth in an unyielding medium like bone and this effect is enhanced, a possible explanation for the relatively early spread of bone growth by the blood stream, to lung in particular. By analogy it might be thought that

43

brain tumours behave similarly. Although the pressure rises within the skull, cancers of the brain are not prone to spread elsewhere for though it is surrounded by vessels the brain carries comparatively few vessels within its substance. The pressure has its effect upon brain function, as does the direct destruction of normal brain by the growth itself but the milieu for distant spread, which pressure conspires to increase, is missing.

There are some forms of malignancy in which no central primary focus of growth can be identified – those affecting the white blood cells. The quality of malignancy of the leukaemias is only represented by the vigour of the malignant cells themselves. The proper place for white cells is within the circulation or the attached filter beds provided by liver or spleen. There can therefore be no question of containment since the habitat of the malignant white cell is the circulation itself. The range of malignancy is wide causing death in a year or less at its worst – usually seen in the young – or simmering on under drug control in a state of symbiosis in the elderly. Yet these cells do not have quite the invasive quality of other tissue cancers. They do not often implant and create new islands of growth, metastases as they are called. They do not take over in other tissues, other than liver and spleen which enlarge with leukaemic infiltration because these organs take part in the formation of white cells. The bone marrow provides cells from which the mature white cell is derived; these are similarly affected, in fact it is at these parent cells that the malignant change occurs. In a sense they invade the bone marrow to the exclusion of other cells produced there for the blood – red cells and platelets, which are less than cells and are particles important for blood clotting. So in leukaemia anaemia develops in two ways. The production of red cells falls. The platelets are responsible for repairing minor defects in the walls of the

44

blood vessels, particularly the small capillaries. These, too, are reduced and red cells tend to leak out into tissue from the surface of intestine, lung or urinary system.

In the same pathological class is lymphosarcoma, a rare disease which affects the lymph nodes rather than the circulating lymphocyte. This does show a tendency to local invasiveness for it starts in tissue which is fixed and does not circulate, though later abnormal lymphocytes are usually seen in circulation.

Hodgkin's disease, lymphadenoma, is another of the white cell malignancies representing a half-way house between the common cancers and leukaemia, for it is in effect a lesion of the lymphoid tissue, of the lymph nodes that is, which enlarge like other cancerous tissues but at first in a discrete way without obviously invading the neighbourhood. This can come later as can implantation, presumably by circulating cells, in organs distant from the affected lymph glands. As in leukaemia the degree of malignancy is variable; it can last as long as fifteen to twenty years before prevailing and the outlook has recently been improved by new drugs, which applied early may hold the disorder in check indefinitely. Lymphadenoma shows less tendency to local invasion from the lymph node in which it starts than lymphosarcoma.

The power of malignant penetration, and therefore the outlook, is a compound of many variables, so much so that precise prediction is not possible in any one individual. In certain organs such as the stomach it is likely to be bad; the gullet likewise. But at some sites, such as the skin, and in some forms growths are so benign as hardly to constitute a cancer in its accepted and dreaded form. Above all is the response of the host to the cancer. Once formed a cancer does not necessarily grow persistently and inexorably in simple or geometric progression. It can remain quiescent for long periods or even regress. For cancer cells are by no means omnipotent; they have to compete with defensive cells in the host, cells which are probably responsible for the destruction of many cancer cells shed into the blood stream – many more circulating cancer cells can be seen than ever succeed in finding a bed successfully to implant in. This resistance is an immunological phenomenon recognized only in recent years. It presents us with great therapeutic problems – how to destroy the cancer cell and not destroy the immunological response in doing so. This is the crux which is only now beginning to occupy our efforts and research and will continue to do so for the rest of this century; this crux will be considered in greater detail anon (Chapter Seven).

CHAPTER FIVE

The Effects of Cancer

The cancer cell contributes nothing to the body's economy. This is not to say that it has no effect. Obviously a tumour by its very nature as a swelling taking up space where no swelling should be, must have some effect. This may impede or impair function in some way depending upon the ease or difficulty with which it can be accommodated. In areas where tissue is lax this space-occupying mass will have little effect. Where there is little room to spare, as in the skull for instance, space for the tumour can only be found at cost to normal structures therein. And there are other ways in which a growth alters function in a purely mechanical or physical sense. Take for example bone.

Bone is the essential scaffold upon which we are built. In our limbs the long bones of arm, forearm, thigh and leg not only support us but with the numerous muscles attached to them allow movement in addition to support. They are really tubes just like our modern scaffolding designed and erected on hard calcareous material to give maximum strength with minimum weight. If they were solid we should have too great a load to carry and the bones would also have less strength. The ends are rounded off into bearings and covered with smooth cartilage to reduce friction in the joints – just like modern bearings with nylon discs inserted for the same purpose. So each long bone has broader bulbous ends connected by shafts. To the shafts the muscles are attached, while the ends are enclosed within the joints, where a little lubrication is

47

provided from the lining – synovia as it is called. Growth in the long bones is cunningly contrived from the ends of the shafts where they meet the bulbous ends of the whole bone itself; for the joints must function during development and it would be difficult to maintain this while growth by simple elongation took place at its ends – as might seem natural. So cellular activity is greatest at these growing areas, at the junction of shaft with end.

Not unexpectedly, therefore, this is a site for cancer. The bone grows from a plate of cartilage; a tumour may, though very rarely, arise here – a chondroma if it is benign, a chondrosarcoma if it is malignant. This produces a mass which as it gets bigger inevitably limits movement at the joint near by. Just one mechanical effect of a tumour in bone.

More common than this, though still rare, is cancer arising from bone cells themselves, also with a tendency to develop near that active growing plate but on the shaft side a little farther away from the joint or at another site of activity just under a membrane, periosteum, which surrounds the shaft and provides cells from which bone develops to increase the girth of the scaffold tube. The cancer is now an osteosarcoma. It does not, as might be expected, improve the strength of the structure. Quite the reverse for as the cells lose their identity and become less well differentiated (Chapter Four) so they lose their hardness and their architectural pattern. So the osteosarcoma bears no semblance of bone order and the shaft becomes soft; the physical structure is disturbed, its strength is lost and in fact the bone may actually break at the tumour.

But these are rare cancers for bone is formed from mesothelium (Chapter Two). Nevertheless cancer within bone is not so very uncommon in late or advanced disease due to spread via the blood stream from commoner growths arising in epithelium elsewhere – breast for example. These secondary growths – metastases – may even announce their presence by fracture of the bone. Metastases from cancer of the breast are less often seen in long bones than in the vertebrae, the bones of the spine – twenty-four of them in all if one excludes the tail bones which have become modified to provide part of the pelvis and are in fact the dovetail joining spine to pelvis. The vertebrae are discs of bone an inch or more thick at the lower end of the spine, less at the top, which can rotate or bend forward and side to side upon one another except in the chest. The twelve vertebrae in the chest are rather limited as regards bending forwards or backwards by the ribs attached to them in order to create the cage around the elastic lungs which are thus enabled to expand and recoil as is necessary for breathing.

Metastases in the spine from breast cancer, when they occur, tend to lodge in the larger lower vertebrae. These carry the weight of the head, chest and abdomen. Since the centre of gravity of the body lies in front of the spine, as the affected vertebrae soften they crumble and collapse in wedge fashion. To be accurate each vertebra is more than a thick disc for attached behind this is an arch of bone. The numerous arches as they are assembled together form a conduit for the telegraph wires to and from the brain, the spinal cord. As in any main trunking system, electrical, telegraphic or what you will, connections run off at intervals to provide terminal supply. So the nerves run out from the spinal cord at regular intervals a pair between each arch, one to the left the other to the right. Failure of the main part of a vertebra will in consequence bring the adjacent arches closer, sometimes so close that these nerves become nipped, particularly on movement of the spine. Thus cancer in the bones of the spine, while it causes little structural defect other than some deformity of its natural curves, can lead to pain through pressure on a nerve.

So function is in no way enhanced by a growth in the structural tissues; quite the reverse. Whether it be in bone or muscle neither are strengthened thereby; the bone may break or collapse, the muscle (very rarely affected by tumours of its own or by metastases) does not contract more powerfully. At the joints mobility may be lost.

But what of the effects in epithelium (Chapter Two) which provides surfaces, linings and secretory glands? In the body's biological economy surfaces and linings are inextricably bound up with secretion. Even the skin secretes its sweat and sebum, an oily protective fluid; rare and relatively benign tumours compromise these glands. It is, however, in the secreting epithelium of other sites, the gut, the lungs and the like, that cancer is common; and it never produces effective secretion. The gastric juice of a man with stomach cancer is not more acid; nor does it contain more pepsin – the digestive juice provided by the stomach. Farther along the alimentary tract the small intestine secretes greatly; but cancer here is very rare and when it occurs it does not secrete. However, some growths of the large intestine do appear to produce mucus. Since mucus secretion and water absorption are the two main functions of this area it might be thought that this represents an attempt at function, but this seems unlikely. We know little about the purpose of mucus for it is a highly complex biochemical field which has hardly been explored; but we do know that there are many molecular computations in mucus giving rise to many varieties. At some time in the not too distant future the activity of mucus, or a multiplicity of activities more probably, will be revealed. In our ignorance we have simply ascribed to mucus the function of lubrication. Mucus is sometimes noticeable when we open our bowels, in a thin layer as though to ease the passage of the faeces. Vaginal mucus is obvious at times clearly to lubricate that passage. Yet mucus is so complex a chemical that it must have required considerable evolutionary effort to attain. Its daily production calls for involved chemistry. Such is biological economy and design, it is improbable that a single purpose is the outcome of all this, unless perhaps mucus is a vestigial chemical remnant, analogous to the appendix, useful at some age in the past when we were on the way to becoming man, but no longer so. The product of a mucus secreting growth is possibly abnormal and since we do not know the functions of normal mucus it is not possible at this moment to know whether or not abnormal mucus induces change by deprivation, by altered action, or any change at all.

It is ironical that a stomach growth is not active in terms of gastric function, for cancer in another organ, the pancreas, can make the stomach work overtime. The pancreas is responsible for several things: it produces digestive enzymes passed in simple fashion through a duct into the duodenum which is the very first part of the intestine after the stomach. But the pancreas also has other secretory cells which do not connect with any ducting system.

In fact there are two distinct mechanisms as regards secretion. Where this is required in a hollow organ, the chemicals for digestion in the gut for instance, the necessary substances, enzymes, are formed in secretory cells grouped together as little glands from which ducts convey the enzymes into the digestive tubes. We can see how this works in the stomach, the essential function of which is to start the process of digestion. Digestive juice is created in the many glands of its lining and flows down ducts into the cavity of the stomach; all the juice has to go to one place where it can be mixed with food, so ducts are appropriate.

There is a large field of secretion which has nothing to

do with digestion. The cells in this group have no ducts, their purpose is to initiate and indeed control function in other cells and organs. They produce in effect chemical messengers – hormones (Chapter Three). There are innumerable cells of this type each with a different function, each producing a specific hormone designed to organize a clearly defined activity. For bodily activity is entirely under biochemical control in every respect. Even the little electrical currents in the nervous system are triggered off by biochemical activity at the nerve junctions. The secretion of digestive enzymes into the stomach is switched on by hormones. The chemicals which switch on this secretion must be delivered to the millions of secretory gland cells with expedition and in a manner which will allow synchronization. Ducting especially designed for this purpose would be quite out of the question so the blood stream is used instead. And this is the paramount distinction of this system of hormonal secretion generally: that the blood stream carries the substance to trigger off activity when it encounters its target.

To return to the pancreas: this organ functions through both systems, passing digestive enzymes through its duct to the duodenum and also possessing several types of hormone secreting cells each with a different purpose. Insulin is the best known of these, the hormone which regulates the sugar in our blood, loss of which leads to diabetes. But there are others, one controlling gastric function, another intestinal activity in a manner as yet not fully understood. A rare tumour sometimes benign, sometimes malignant, can develop from the cells controlling gastric secretion. These tumour cells remain well differentiated (Chapter Four) and retain their function with the result that the gastric secretory cells are kept in a high state of activity. Much more hydrochloric acid is produced than is required and repeated ulceration of stomach and duodenum develops. So while a cancer of the stomach itself is functionally inactive, a growth in the pancreas may cause increased gastric activity.

While the pancreas is a gland possessing both forms of secretion, there are glands like the thyroid which are totally ductless. Oddly, while tumours of ducted glands appear not to function, growths of ductless glands can be biologically active depending upon the degree of differentiation of the cancer cell, the more malignant the less likely the cells will be active in this way. A growth of the insulin cells of the pancreas will be productive causing the individual to be short of sugar in the blood; of the gastrin producing cell will cause the stomach to secrete more acid but a cancer of the pancreatic cells which produce a digestive juice is inactive and no more of this is turned out – quite the reverse. So it is generally: tumours of ductless glands can and often do secrete; the others do not.

The hormones produced in tumours are usually normal to that gland; though normal, their effect is physiologically abnormal for the excess available creates distortion. The thyroid is responsible for our temperature control. In a sense it is like a thermostat and activity regulator rolled into one for it controls the rate at which we burn our fuel. Thus it controls our temperature and ordains the rate of activity of our cells. We slow down in every way when the thyroid fails as it sometimes does, though more often it is the other way round. Increased activity of the thyroid, hyperthyroidism, is not uncommon; the patient feels hot, sweats, is jumpy and his pulse rate and temperature increase. Mostly the origin of this condition has nothing to do with cancer at all. Nevertheless some cancers of the thyroid can produce the relevant secretion, thyroxin, and so display activity. However this is seldom, for the cells of most thyroid cancers are not sufficiently differentiated from their normal brothers (Chapter Four) to be active.

The adrenal is a multipurpose ductless gland; cancer can affect any one of its numerous different cells and produce results which differ widely depending upon the cell type involved. It may be high blood pressure or a variety of other conditions which can on the one hand change the body's configuration, on the other its sexual characteristics.

The testis and the ovary have dual function but are not quite like the pancreas. Both are ductless glands producing respectively androgen, the male hormone, or oestrogen, the female equivalent. In addition the testis has a duct system to carry sperms to the reservoir designed for their containment until released, the seminal vesicles. Likewise the ovary, though oddly the duct to carry the ovum to the uterus falls short of the ovary itself. So the ovum has to make its way across a part of the abdominal cavity (Chapter Four) to gain access into its tube. Sometimes an ovum miscarries and sperms come up the tube, out into the abdominal cavity to meet it, so that an embryo develops outside the womb. But this is unusual and not part of our story. As regards cancer of these two organs sperms and ova are not affected; no monsters are produced. Hormonal function is rarely brought into play by cancer and then only in growths of the ovary.

Cancer may therefore make itself felt by the activity of its cells – a primary effect; but this appears to be confined to tumours of the ductless glands and these are uncommon in the total field of cancer. The effects of cancer and so its symptoms and presentation are most commonly secondary phenomena – anaemia, for instance, due simply to persistent blood loss from an ulcerated surface, for cancers at the inner surfaces of organs and when they reach the skin become ulcerated.

For the most part cancer presents itself by impingement either of the tumour itself on the affected organ or upon organs near by, or of its seedlings in a similar way.

54

Essentially this brings about physical effects which are not difficult to understand or predict. A hollow tube-like organ such as the intestine will tend to become blocked after an initial period of very variable duration, possibly months, sometimes years. During this interval an ulcerated surface of relatively small dimension, an inch or two across, is the only phenomenon which might give rise to symptoms, such as anaemia, and often to none. The small intestine is a very rare site for cancer, but in the large intestine it is not uncommon. When blockage and obstruction supervene, albeit gradually, the symptoms are those which common sense would suggest, namely alteration in bowel habit gradually leading to colic and distension with ultimate failure to open the bowels or pass wind.

At the other end of the alimentary tract is the oesophagus, the tube connecting mouth with stomach. When this becomes blocked the patient has difficulty in swallowing, causing a sense of food sticking in one place. At the same time weight is rapidly lost for, in contrast with a large intestinal lesion, insufficient food reaches those areas of the intestine designed for digestion and absorption.

It is not difficult to see that the effects of a growth of the stomach must be similar since this is only one step onwards from the oesophagus. Yet the symptom pattern is different for, though weight is lost, first loss of appetite and then vomiting predominate with the addition of the sort of pain we all associate with indigestion or vomiting. The oesophagus has the sole function of passing food from mouth to the areas which bring about digestion; the predominant symptom is therefore difficulty in swallowing. But the stomach acts both as reservoir and a mill for mincing and preparing food for digestion to be completed lower down. Much fluid is secreted through the stomach wall and this is lost through vomiting.

These are direct effects from impingement and blockage.

The pancreas is an organ where a tumour most often declares itself by second hand, through its effect on another organ. Cancer of its ductless cells is very rare; more commonly a growth develops in the other cells which manufacture enzymes for the digestion of fat and protein. These may be reduced, or even lost through blockage of the main pancreatic duct, the diameter of which is no greater than a pencil lead. But the effect is slight since other enzymes in the small intestine almost complete the pancreatic task. Unless and until the cancer invades the abdominal wall behind it, thus causing pain, the tumour tends to remain symptomatically silent. However, the main canal which carries bile from the liver into the gut passes, as though by chance, through the pancreas. A tumour of the pancreas growing near by will eventually press upon the bile duct and stop the flow from the liver. The bile is dammed back and there is nowhere for it to go except into the blood vessels of the liver. It breaks through into these and circulates in the blood; its yellow pigments then cause jaundice. So cancer of one part of the pancreas can, by its propinquity to this duct, be one of the causes of jaundice. And at the same time, because these pigments normally colour the contents of the intestine, their diversion away from the gut leaves the faeces, as they emerge, pale, almost white in colour. Meanwhile the urine darkens because the pigments circulating in the blood pass through that filter, the kidney, and are excreted in the urine. However, cancer is only one of the causes of obstruction to normal bile outflow. Nobody who develops jaundice should infer that they must have cancer. Some may have, the majority have not, even though seedlings from growths starting elsewhere sometimes lodge in the liver and obstruct the bile duct by pressure where it runs through and out of the liver.

There are pathological processes other than cancer itself which may be brought in train by the presence of a growth.

Inflammation is one. This is a reaction within any tissue, initiated by the body in response to damage. It is protective and starts off the chain of events leading to repair. You scratch yourself; inflammation immediately follows. Bacterial invasion, infection that is, elicits the inflammatory response. Cancers can be associated with infection in two ways. Many grow at a surface or as they enlarge reach it; there they ulcerate – on the skin or on an inner surface such as the gut or urinary bladder. Bacteria are present at these surfaces, ordinarily held harmlessly at bay by the normal surface cells. But when these cells are breached the bacteria can take root in the ulcer. This is 'secondary' infection, secondary to the malignant lesion. Inflammation follows. Pus, the product of the inflammatory reaction, may exude, and because swelling of tissue is also part of inflammation, tenderness and pain may arise from the tissues surrounding the growth as they become inflamed.

Infection is also prone to occur when the normal flow of secretion is impeded. Thus a hold up in the stream of urine from kidney to bladder encourages infection. Returning to the pancreas: a tumour growing not sufficiently close to the bile duct to cause jaundice, may yet have an obstructive effect upon the main pancreatic duct causing inflammation in the gland behind the obstruction and so pain. Here the dammed-up secretions set off inflammation by digesting the tissues which created them.

In the lungs the situation is different. The bronchi conduct air into the lungs where oxygen can diffuse into the blood through the thin lung wall. A growth blocking a bronchus leads to collapse of part of the lung, but in terms of lung function the growth has little direct effect. Though the area of lung beyond the growth cannot be ventilated once the lesion has blocked the passage to it, much spare capacity for oxygenation of the blood remains elsewhere in the chest. Even a lobe of one lung, which would ordinarily undertake one-fifth or so of the total respiratory work, can be lost to circuit without noticeable change, though some breathlessness may ensue. But more often the symptoms of lung cancer reflect the fact that infection tends to supervene where a normal passageway is blocked or partially blocked. So a patient with lung cancer develops sputum with pus and often a little blood and a cough. Pain may be felt when the lining surrounding the lung (the pleura referred to in Chapter Four) is involved either by the growth or the secondary infection and inflammation. Then an effusion of fluid may form in the potential cavity between the pleura on the lung and the pleura lining the chest wall around it. As this space fills with fluid so lung tissue beyond the original area and otherwise normal becomes compressed, leading to further respiratory embarrassment. Diagnosis in these circumstances is not easily come by for lung cancer more often affects those with pre-existing lung disease; they already have breathlessness and a cough producing purulent sputum so that the development of a cancer strikes no warning note.

Cancer at these sites has been selected to exemplify the way the disease brings about its effects. A simple knowledge of human function and form, even indeed of biology, will indicate the possible results of development of a tumour elsewhere. Inside the skull the effects will result from destruction of the area involved, from pressure on nerves emerging near by or from blockage to the flow of the fluid which bathes it and passes on oxygen and nutrition from the blood. In this respect brain differs from other tissues such as muscle with a more direct supply from the blood.

A special system contains this fluid which flows over and around the surface of the brain and the nerve tissue running from it down the duct in the spine. It actually passes inside the brain through a little hole into hollow cisterns within each half of the brain. The fluid is secreted within the brain and flows outwards through the hole. This anatomical arrangement is vulnerable for the small hole can become blocked so that fluid formed in the brain is trapped. Secretion continues and, though infection does not supervene here, the pressure tends to rise. In fact some babies are born with an anomaly – the hole remains imperforate. Fluid accumulates within the brain – hydrocephalus when translated into the technical jargon of medicine. In the baby this is noticeable because the bones of the skull have not yet fused into the complete carapace which forms the intact skull enclosing and protecting the brain within. As the tension inside the brain rises the component bones are pushed apart and the whole head gets larger.

Not so in the adult, whose skull is rigid. A growth can distort the approaches to the hole if near enough or may close it directly but the skull does not give way with the increasing pressure inside it and so there is no enlargement of the head. Instead the internal tension produces symptoms. Headache, vomiting and eventually mental confusion occur. If nerves are disturbed by pressure or invasion of the tumour weaknesses will appear, often in the eyes or face: or sensation will be lost. All must depend upon the site of the growth. For example a not very malignant growth affects nerves from the ear; it will disturb hearing on that side and, in addition, certain other nerves together with those parts of the brain which lie adjacent. Since the tumour develops well to the outside of the brain pressure increases only after a considerable interval and will only do so when the tumour is of sufficient size to create considerable distortion and displacement within the skull. Meanwhile weakness may be noticed in the face or in movements of the eye, since

59

adjacent nerves carry this function; or unsteadiness of gait and inco-ordinated action supervene because that part of the brain responsible for such control is close by.

Tumours arising from brain substance project symptoms similar to those which arise from the membranes interposed between skull and brain. Though the result in terms of symptoms can be the same the significance may, however, be very different, for growths of brain tissue are invasively malignant, whereas the others are muted in this respect, their capacity being to recur at their original site if some of the original cells remain after removal has been attempted.

But many a brain tumour in its earlier days lies sequestered in an area where pressure effects on nerves or the flow of fluid are not brought into play; so it remains unnoticed. Moreover, unlike other cancers, tumours within the skull show little inclination to disseminate and seed elsewhere, probably reflecting the fewer blood vessels and the absence of lymphatics within the skull.

The potential for spread is great in stomach cancer because it is well endowed with blood and lymph; it seeds in liver and lung. Any growth of the intestine can likewise pass to liver because of the special arrangements of the blood supply necessary to carry all the products of digestion for processing there. The kidney, though also within the abdomen, has no reason to pass blood to the liver; its seedlings, its metastases, are borne by the blood directly to lung and elsewhere while local lymph nodes at the back of the abdomen are also involved.

As the ripples widen and other distant sites are involved in the wash, so accretions are added to the symptomatic picture, so the disabilities change and increase. Metastases are the manifestation of blood transport; though they can develop anywhere there is a predilection for the lung, which one must surmise acts as a filter of finer mesh than other organs, in which the little floating groups of malignant cells can become enmeshed. The total volume of the blood passes through the lungs in one circulation; other organs only take their share of what comes their way. For the lung has to process each and every red cell, whereas it is only necessary for the kidney, for example, to tap the main blood supply in order to draw off fluid to be processed, to be cleared of waste, and to attract enough red cells to provide its own oxygen requirement. So the lung is at particular risk from the aggregations of cells which break off from a malignancy. A metastasis in the lung, or metastases since they are usually multiple, will clearly produce results similar to those of a growth which starts there.

The turnover of blood through the heart is no less than in the lungs, so it may seem odd that metastases do not settle here, or at the most very rarely indeed. A moment's reflection provides a possible answer for in addition to the fact that cancer cells rarely implant in muscle, here the blood flows as a torrent and it is physically as difficult for seedlings to settle as it is for water weeds in a cascade. Indeed the rare metastases that do grow in the heart most probably get there through the heart's own blood supply and did not settle from within the agitated chambers of the pump itself.

So the lung and liver are the organs most commonly involved in metastatic deposition. Indeed it is through secondary deposits at these sites that a cancer may first become manifest. Often the original tumour where the cancerous process began gives rise to no symptoms and its presence is only declared by the development of the seedling growths elsewhere. The cellular change of malignancy may cause no general disturbance nor local destruction. This poses two problems in the control of cancer. It is impossible to know when a growth started its life or how long it has remained in abeyance. It is also difficult to ascertain evidence of its presence at an early stage.

A simplistic view prevails that cancer spreads progressively, at first being confined, then finding its way along lymphatics – local spread – and finally disseminating widely; an ordered progression, in fact. If this were so early treatment would be effective and the earlier the better. Orderliness is certainly true of skin cancer in all its forms, but unlikely in many of the other common cancers such as breast, where dissemination through the blood stream may take place before local spread, though this is not to say that it always does. On the orthodox philosophy of orderliness is based the concept of the 'early' case and the propaganda encouraging patients to report mild and early symptoms to their doctor. But early in this sense means reporting to the doctor as soon as symptoms are noticed. The onset of symptoms bears no certain relationship to the actual state of affairs as regards the growth. One growth may take years before making its presence felt, another may do so in considerably less time. It all depends upon the nature of the beast and where it is placed. Herein lies confusion which still bedevils accurate assessment and efficient treatment.

CHAPTER SIX

Investigation and Diagnosis

The first step in the care of a patient, whatever may be wrong, is to find out what is wrong. A glimpse of the obvious, perhaps. This should come before treatment though it does not always do so. For by diagnosis is meant to 'know thoroughly'. In medical terms this necessitates finding the pathological cause and the extent of the disease. It is not enough to recognize, for example, that someone is suffering from intestinal obstruction; which is really a condition and not a disease – a condition, in fact, of failure of dynamics in an important system in the body. For diagnosis we need to know the cause in terms of the disease which has given rise to the obstruction. Only when we know the disease can the outlook be assessed with any accuracy and effective treatment be applied.

Diagnosis is therefore the imperative immediate aim but it cannot always be achieved before treatment has to be applied. The gut is hidden within the abdomen; often the cause of its obstruction can only be inferred from a number of signs and possibilities. It cannot be known thoroughly. Nevertheless the situation is so urgent that operation must be undertaken before the surgeon can be sure of the cause. Treatment and the moment of diagnosis may coincide for the surgeon is likely to see the cause when he opens the abdomen to relieve the obstruction. But he may not; for what he sees he may not be able to recognize and identify. Diagnosis will then await the closer examination under the microscope by a pathologist of any particle of tissue the surgeon may be able to remove. And even the pathologist is sometimes nonplussed. So diagnosis can be elusive.

This is only one example of the need for action without being sure quite where one is going. It happens in many aspects of acute medicine. Some infections can develop suddenly and with such severity that an antibiotic has to be given before the bacteria causing the infection is known, in the hope that this will strike lucky. It could be argued that a diagnosis has been made when infection or intestinal obstruction has been pronounced. But these are part of the knowledge we need, not the whole. Diagnosis in its proper sense is needed for full and proper understanding and management of any case; and the earlier the better.

This basic tactic of medicine, to try to discover the diagnosis first, applies to cancer as much as any other disease. It is not enough in cancer simply to know that the disease is present; nor is there any test which will reveal this. It would be an achievement if such could be found – a sample of blood, perhaps, which on analysis showed changes in its composition indicating that cancer is present somewhere, a test which would be made at regular intervals. Much effort is being made to find one. But when the effort succeeds, as it will, we shall still be left with finding the site.

As yet we have no such test so diagnostic endeavour starts from the onset of symptoms. It is seldom that a diagnosis can be conclusive at this stage, though the symptoms may be highly suggestive. On examination of the patient the discovery of a swelling may be almost conclusive, in the breast, the abdomen or the limbs – in any part of the body that is accessible to the palpating hand; or meets the eye because it is on the surface. Tumours growing within the chest and skull are inaccessible to ordinary examination as are some parts of the abdomen. Other means of demonstrating them are necessary.

64

Recourse is then had to diagnostic X-rays. A beam of X-rays can be shone through the body on to a photographic plate. The beam is impeded to a greater or lesser extent by the nature of the tissue it passes through. Bone, containing the heavy element calcium, absorbs more X-rays than soft tissue. So a silhouette appears in the photograph with the bones showing up light and the rest darker where the negative has been more exposed to the X-rays. The soft tissue itself shows some degree of contrast depending on its thickness. Thus it is possible to discern the 'shadow' of the liver or a kidney. Indeed the time of the exposure can be varied, just as in any photograph. By shortening the exposure penetration with X-rays is reduced thus improving contrast between different soft tissues.

X-ray diagnosis is applicable in two ways. The straightforward approach is a direct photograph. If a tumour is present in the lungs it will show on the film because it is solid and so is more dense than the air-containing sacs around it. Not so, however, with growths in the stomach or bowel for the tissue around the tumour is solid. Something else has to be done. Since the gut is a conduit all that is necessary is to introduce a material which will absorb the X-rays. This will then show up the inner outline of whatever part of the gut is under investigation. If a growth is present it will either impinge as a swelling or cause a stricture, both of which will be demonstrated as an irregularity of outline by the dense, radio-opaque, medium. A suspension of barium sulphate is used; it is insoluble and so will not be absorbed. It is given either by mouth in the form of a barium meal which will display the gullet, stomach and small intestine; or by barium enema for demonstration of the large intestine.

More sophisticated methods are necessary for showing up the kidney or the gall bladder for the radio-opaque material cannot be introduced easily into these organs. There is an inherent advantage in what at first appears to be a disadvantage. Soluble materials, usually containing an iodine compound, are used; these are selectively secreted by the organ under investigation. A radio-opaque 'dye' can be given by mouth which is absorbed in the stomach and duodenum, then passes to the liver and thus into the bile. It becomes concentrated in the gall bladder which then shows up by contrast against its surroundings when the X-ray is taken. However, concentration only takes place in the gall bladder so something stronger is required if the ducts running from the liver to the gall bladder and on from there are to be demonstrated. For this purpose an injection into a vein is used. Yet another material is introduced into the blood stream for revealing the kidneys.

The advantage of this method lies not only in the fact that the outline of the organ can be seen but also that its function may be assessed. One kidney may show delay in excretion of the dye, or both; for it is known how soon the dye should appear after injection when kidney function is normal. The disadvantages are twofold, for the contrast is never so strong when excretion or secretion methods are used so that the resulting picture is not so clear cut. And if the disorder has caused the organ to stop working nothing will be seen; then the only information gained is that the organ is out of action. It is not possible to discern why it does not work – whether a tumour is blocking it or whether it has been destroyed by some other disease.

If the gall bladder fails to function there is nothing more to be done, but in the case of the kidney there is. An instrument called a cystoscope can be passed up into the urinary bladder. It is an ingenious piece of engineering comprising a telescope, a light at its inner end and small fine controls which enable certain manœuvres to be undertaken within the bladder by remote control. Through

66

the telescope the organ can be inspected and the openings of the little pipes which lead to it from the kidneys can be seen. If a growth is present in the bladder it will be observed. At the same time fine flexible tubes, no more than a millimetre or two in thickness, can be guided into the ureters (that is the pipes from the kidney) to permit the injection of contrast medium – the radio-opaque dye.

Air acts in negative contrast to soft tissue and its disposition in the gut shown up on an ordinary X-ray of the abdomen is sometimes informative particularly when the intestines are obstructed. In obstruction fluid is retained as well as air the two forming a contrasting interface; the tell-tale fluid levels then indicate that a blockage is present.

Air is injected intentionally to create contrast in the brain where it will fill the cisterns (Chapter Five) so that the denser brain tissue stands out against the background of air and asymmetry of one of its lobes can be discerned. This is done by an injection into the lower part of the back through into the spine (Chapter Five) whence it can float upwards to the brain. Radio-opaque material can be used in this way to show up the spinal cord but this method is now only used very rarely since this substance has been known to cause reaction in the delicate nervous tissue and the membranes which surround it.

In recent years contrast using the blood stream has been widely developed particularly for the display of deep-seated tumours. The blood vessels pursue a constant course because the structure of the body as a whole – where all the organs lie and their juxtapositions – is almost entirely constant from one individual to another. This is a fact of life: that the structure and relationships of the organs of the body of a species of any moving creature will be the same from one individual to another. In contrast the structure of living things rooted to the ground they grow from only follows a general plan showing wide variations from one individual to another. Even the number of limbs in a tree is variable.

The anatomy of man has been known in detail for centuries and can be learnt as a three-dimensional map by medical students. Even the arteries follow a known and certain course and their final branches at each organ provide a pattern special to that organ. The presence of a tumour disturbs that pattern both by displacement and the fact that it develops its own blood supply. So a radio-opaque dye injected into an artery appropriately placed for delivery to the organ in question will reveal an abnormality of pattern and of flow. Not only this. In developing its own blood supply the tumour tends to outline itself and at the same time by pressure on surrounding tissue obliterates the normal flow around it, leaving a clearer zone there. Angiography, as this is called, which started as a means of demonstrating disease in arteries themselves, has now found a valuable application in the detection of cancer.

This technique has been extended to the lymphatics (Chapter Four) and provides two pieces of information: whether the flow in the lymphatics is reduced or actually reversed by obstruction and the size and consistency of the lymph nodes themselves. For the spread of cancer to these nodes and cancer which starts within them will tend to impede the flow of lymph. There are many lymph channels so that the fluid, when dammed back at a node will flow back and around elsewhere. The node itself will either appear obliterated on the X-ray photograph, or, if some lymph gains access to it, it will be seen to be enlarged.

Obviously the diagnosis of cancer is easiest come by if it can be seen. So methods have been devised to extend vision beyond the surface. Cystoscopy has already been mentioned. There are numerous other 'scopes' designed to pass through orifices: through the mouth down into the gullet (the oesophagoscope), on into the stomach (the gastroscope), or into the larynx and the windpipes (the laryngoscope and the bronchoscope); from below up into the large bowel (the sigmoidoscope). It is even possible to make a small incision in the skin and pass a peritoneoscope into the abdominal cavity and look at the surface of organs there. Most of these instruments are simpler than the cystoscope for they can be wider and so permit direct vision. The peritoneoscope is like the cystoscope but the gastroscope is more complex for the stomach is shaped like a J, creating the need to look round corners. This is achieved by making the instrument flexible, the lens system being created out of bundles of very fine nylon threads along which 'cold' light can be shone and the object seen with magnification despite the bends.

By thus bringing more to the eye, more is also brought to hand. It is usually possible to diagnose a cancer by sight but it is helpful to be doubly sure. So whenever possible a small piece of the offending tissue is taken to be scrutinized under the microscope. This is known as a biopsy. Biopsy is possible through any scope. Not infrequently it is undertaken as a separate small operation under local anaesthetic when a lymph node is enlarged, to see whether it contains cancer. Smears taken from the cervix of the womb are a form of biopsy and for many years samples from within the womb itself have been obtained by means of a small operation. Blood samples are yet another form of biopsy, in this circumstance being used for looking at the blood cells to diagnose leukaemia. Sometimes it is necessary to carry this further and obtain some of the blood forming cells from the bone marrow, and this can be done by inserting a strong needle into the centre of the breast bone.

There are parts of the body where the evidence of cancer may be hard to come by. The liver is a case in point:

69

It is true that a needle can be inserted into the liver through the abdominal wall to obtain a small core of tissue for inspection under the microscope and if cancer, usually spread from elsewhere, is widespread in the liver then the necessary evidence will be brought to light. But if there are only one or two deposits the needle may well miss them. For these circumstances there is another method increasingly coming into use employing radioactive materials. It is only necessary to find a suitable substance known to be taken up and handled by the organ under scrutiny and then make some part of it radioactive. This is usually given to the patient by mouth but may be injected. The radioactivity it emits can then be perceived through a special receiver which scans the area overlying the organ. A map is drawn which will show either areas of increased or decreased uptake by contrast against the general background of uptake in the organ. A growth in the liver will appear as a negative shadow against the rest. Where the cells of a tumour continue to function as sometimes occurs in any ductless gland (Chapter Five) the growth will be displayed in the opposite way; scanning will reveal a greater deposition of the radioactive material there than elsewhere.

By various means the full diagnosis is built up. The symptoms, and the examination of the patient which follows therefrom, may suffice to indicate that a swelling is cancer and not something else. In order to be sure a biopsy may have to be taken. But this is insufficient to know thoroughly. Whether or not spread has occurred, and if so how far, is all part of the diagnosis in cancer. Thus the investigations, or some of them, may be needed for this purpose. An X-ray photograph of the chest is almost routinely taken since the lungs are a likely site for seedlings to settle and grow. Scanning is in its infancy but as it becomes established so the liver, for the same reason, should become a site for this investigation whenever a cancer in the intestines or stomach is suspected.

In addition there is the microscopic examination of a biopsy or the growth itself after it has been removed. For from this is learnt the nature of the growth and also its cellular behaviour, whether it is well-differentiated or otherwise (Chapter Four).

Only when all this information has been gathered is it possible to prognosticate – perhaps the most important act in medicine. Above all we wish to know what will become of us; an occasional individual when he is ill may not, but his relations will. And this can only be achieved by weighing numerous factors – the growth, its type, how far it has gone, the age and personality of the patient and the state of his health generally. He may have a heart condition which could preclude operation and so limit the choice of treatment. So further investigations may be required unrelated to the cancer and designed to reveal general fitness; whether amongst other things anaemia is present so that this may be corrected and operation be performed more safely. And against all this has to be set the effectiveness of the varieties of treatment.

CHAPTER SEVEN

Treatment

The strategy of treatment is obvious and simple. It must be the removal of the cancer. This can sometimes be achieved by the simple process of surgical excision. A growth that has got no further than its initial site, a growth that is still only a localized tumour from which cells have not spread along the lymphatic canals nor floated into the blood stream can clearly be removed provided it is not placed in or so near to a vital organ that its removal is out of the question. Fortunately surgical ingenuity is such that the chances of removal are seldom limited in this way. Skin cancer is a case in point. Easily encompassed and unlikely to have spread, its excision is nearly always followed by success. If the defect in the skin is too great to be closed by the simple process of drawing the edges of the wound together with stitches, it can be covered with a skin graft. There is no vital organ at stake if the breast has to be removed for a growth there. Much of the intestine can be removed without noticeable effect. Similarly with the lung; and if the kidney is at fault it has its pair on the other side and this has sufficient capacity to take over the work of two.

The task is greater and the outcome less certain when spread is known to have occurred or is likely to have done. It is only lymphatic spread which is amenable to excision, for dissemination by blood stream is so widespread as to make surgical encompassment out of the question. So where the lymph glands are involved as a result of a skin cancer both may be removed. This principle applies in any part of the body, but the outcome will be less successful in organs where the lymph drains away in various directions to numerous lymph nodes, as from the stomach.

Nevertheless to know whether the growth has been encompassed is not as simple as it sounds, for this is a cellular disease and a few cells may be lurking in a lymph node without being noticeable at examination either before or at operation. Why not, then, remove as much lymphatic tissue as possible as a routine when removing a growth with a known propensity to spread? And this is precisely the basis on which cancer surgery has been conducted until now. However, views are changing in this respect – and more of this anon.

The problem of the undetected seedling has also been tackled in another way – by X-rays, and more recently by special chemicals called cytotoxic drugs, a field of treatment which has been developed from – of all things – mustard gas. Irradiation by X-rays in much higher dose than is needed for diagnostic purposes – or other means such as radium or radioactive cobalt – damages the nuclei of all cells so that they die. If concentrated on a tumour this, in effect, should destroy the growth and thus remove it no less effectively than excision – provided all the cells in the tumour succumb. At the same time only a little normal tissue is affected, that tissue which lies close by, for irradiation is like light and can be directed like the beam from a torch. The areas where possible seedlings may be growing can be 'sterilized' thus. So for a long time it has been the practice either to remove a growth surgically and treat the field of possible lymphatic spread by irradiation if accessible to X-rays. For many years the routine treatment for breast cancer comprised both removal of the breast followed by X-ray therapy. In some circumstances the primary growth can be treated very successfully by X-rays alone without operation, cancer of the skin being a case in point. However, though some cancers yield to irradiation, not all do so; some may be almost completely resistant, others partially.

Surgery and X-rays can take no account of cells which have been disseminated throughout the body, most of which die of their own accord leaving the survivors to take root as metastases. Nor can they be effective in those malignant conditions which affect the circulating white cells – the leukaemias. Antibiotics have proved their worth in killing bacteria circulating throughout the body, so by analogy surely it should be possible to find a chemical which will destroy the malignant cell without damaging normal tissues? The pursuit of this panacea has been conducted for some time and there are now a variety of drugs – cytotoxic drugs – which selectively damage malignant cells, but none has yet been found which is fully effective in the way antibiotics have proved themselves to be with bacterial infections. However, the results of cyto-toxic therapy are improving.

Nevertheless treatment for cancer has now reached a state of paradox. The simple approach of excision or ablation is no longer fully tenable. It succeeds with the less malignant forms – many of the skin cancers and indeed those which spread gradually and at first to the lymph nodes and only very late in their existence to the blood stream. Difficulty arises with those growths which disseminate, because of our inability to know whether a growth has already disseminated at the time the patient is first seen: whether, indeed, dissemination occurs early in the life of a cancer or after a latent period. Cancer of the breast is a common growth; its natural history is widely variable. At one end of the scale it appears to remain localized for many years without affecting lymph drainage or becoming evident elsewhere; even without treatment, it

74

may not influence survival. At the other, despite energetic treatment, a growth causes early death through general spread, indeed its course appears to be unimpeded by treatment.

The simplistic view, which has governed our therapeutic endeavours until now, has been based upon the concept of orderliness – that lymph nodes will become involved and thereafter, or even in some minds *then*, the growth will spread elsewhere by the blood stream. But the spread of cancer cells is less likely to be governed by order than by disorder. Whether a growth leaks into the blood stream before moving along the channels of lymph drainage is a matter of chance and the virulence of the cell. The view is gaining ground that dissemination may occur at the outset – and of what avail then excision of the growth and its lymph drainage? Some are even of the opinion that all breast cancers disseminate from the outset; that cancer cells may be found circulating in the blood at any time but that most, and not infrequently all, are destroyed until the time arrives when the dose of cells is greater than can be contained; the body's defences are flooded and overwhelmed.

The paradox is twofold. In the face of uncertainty as regards the extent of the disease and therefore how extensive treatment should be, the treatment itself can encourage the spread of cancer. Irradiation is a potent cause of cancerous change in normal cells. It is used because it is more immediately destructive to the malignant cell nucleus than the normal. But the dose must be carefully controlled if normal tissue is not to undergo change, particularly the blood cells.

It is now beginning to be realized that an operation may reduce the natural defences within the body to cancer invasion. What then are these defences? Evidence has been accumulating that some form of immunity is developed

75

within the body against the cancer cell. Immunity has long been understood in the context of bacterial infection. Such invasion is contained by the larger white blood cells, ingesting the bacteria themselves while their poisons are neutralized by the production of chemicals called antibodies developed especially for this purpose and carried throughout the body in the blood. While this system was being clarified and understood over the centuries which have followed the first use of vaccination by Jesty for smallpox, no evidence was forthcoming that this antibody system played any part in cancer.

However, research undertaken early in this century indicated some reaction to cancer, for tumours transplanted from one animal to another did not take and were rejected. Unfortunately much of this work took no account of the fact that any tissue from one animal, whether cancerous or not, would be rejected by another whether of the same species or not. Graft a piece of skin from a mouse on to a guinea pig or from one guinea pig to another and it will be rejected, that is, it will be cast off after about three weeks even though it will appear to have been united with the host and soundly healed during that period. Moreover, the skin of one man will behave similarly when grafted on to another, even from a parent to a child; but not from one identical twin to another.

This rejection is an immunity response; during the three week period a reaction develops against the foreign cells of the donor. It does not occur in twins because of their genetic identity; they display compatibility in such systems as blood groups. Blood groups are, in fact, a relatively simple example of the situation of immune rejection; for blood transfusion is in effect a graft of red cells and compatibility relies upon the cells of the donor matching the relevant 'antibody' system within the recipient. Whereas in blood grafting the cells encounter a system

76

already in being other tissue cells are not catered for in advance. So why do the cells of a graft always become rejected as do red cells of incompatible blood? Or not quite, because the rejection of red cells is immediate since the antibody is present when transfusion occurs, whereas rejection takes time for grafts – a delayed immunity reaction in fact.

The development of organ transplantation – of kidneys and hearts – and the need therefore to suppress this immunological reaction has intensified study and so enlightened us as regards this type of reaction. It is mediated through the smaller white cells, the lymphocytes. These invade the graft, which is foreign to the individual receiving it because the protein composition of its cells are not identical with those of the host. The complex proteins are incompatible – except, once more, in identical twins who have identical nuclear templates so that any proteins they form are the same. Thus any tissue or organ can be grafted from one twin to its identical pair, but not in unlike twins, in whom compatibility is never complete.

In cancer the cell nucleus has changed, the proteins it produces are therefore foreign to the host, albeit less markedly so than in a graft; so that cancers are in effect foreign, some more markedly so than others. And this is reflected in the microscopic appearances where sometimes infiltration of the cancer with lymphocytes may be seen intermingling with the cancer cell – the biter bit.

So in medical practice today not only has the lymphocyte become a cell of prime importance but the attitude towards it is ambivalent to say the least. If an organ is transplanted the lymphocytes must be suppressed; if a cancer is to be treated they must be encouraged, for they will assist in containment of the growth and attack the cells which float away to form seedlings.

The white cells are more susceptible than other normal

cells in the body both to irradiation and cytotoxic drugs. When treating cancer with X-rays or drugs care is taken to ensure that these cells are not reduced dangerously in number. At the same time any slight impairment of their activity may, for all we know, reduce their effectiveness in the aim we are seeking – the destruction of the cancer. Conversely both X-rays and cytotoxic drugs are used to suppress the lymphocytes in order to maintain a transplanted organ. In this there lies a danger, for cancer may be promoted thereby. It has now been demonstrated that prolonged suppression of lymphocytes in mice leads to the development of cancer. Moreover, there are indications that man himself may react in this way. Quite a number of patients are now living for three years or more with transplanted kidneys. They would not be alive but for the transplant. Nevertheless cancers have developed in some of these patients and only time can tell, as the numbers increase, whether the incidence is higher in them than would ordinarily be expected.

As regards the treatment of cancer the implications of our recent knowledge about lymphocytes is wider. Irradiation and drugs can be detrimental. But so can an operation itself. Clearly the lymphatic system, particularly the lymph nodes, should be preserved. But in the simple terms which have formed the basis of surgical extirpation, terms which still dictate the orthodoxy of our treatment, the growth has to be removed and with it the regional lymph nodes since they present the next area of direct spread – that is spread other than dissemination through the blood stream. It has been standard practice to remove the main drainage area of the breast: the lymph nodes in the armpit whether or not they were involved. Even in recent times removal of breast cancer by exponents of radical surgery caused them to attempt the extreme – removal of the whole lymphatic area of drainage beyond the armpit and

78

also within the chest. So strong has been the principle of 'clearance' of the whole field of possible contamination, whether involved or not, as a general principle of surgery, that it has been almost a matter of negligence not to do so. While there are a few surgeons who still hold this view, many now consider that it cannot be in the patient's interest if all lymph nodes are removed. What, then, if some of these lymph nodes are left behind at operation containing a cancer seedling which could not be detected because it was too small? This is probably a lesser hazard than removing too much lymphatic tissue. The seedling will grow and this can be removed when it becomes apparent later. Moreover, there is no evidence that further seedlings are spread from a metastasis, only from the primary growth itself.

What we are considering is the endeavour to cure. A tumour which has not spread in any way can be cured by removal provided the local anatomy will permit, that its attachment or the organ of its origin is dispensable. For some tumours, particularly surface ones, we can be reasonably sure of cure not only because we can see them and size them up, but from our knowledge of their natural history. Otherwise removal for cure is no more than an attempt, the efficacy of which only time will reveal. Meanwhile we may break the barriers which the lymphatic system provides; indeed we may disseminate the cancer in the very act of excision, for handling a growth is known to increase the number of tumour cells liberated into the blood stream. Many of these blood-borne cells come to naught either because they have not the power to implant or more probably because they are engulfed by the lymphatic cells. And here is another difficulty, for the stress of an operation has now been shown to reduce the capability of lymphatic cells for a period of two or so weeks. Their vitality and power to reproduce is weakened; so that the barrier which may well be effective in sweeping the blood stream clear of the cells ordinarily shed from the tumour is less effective at the time of operation when a greater escape occurs, and for a short time thereafter.

Nevertheless surgery is usually essential for other reasons: in order to relieve symptoms and to avoid and overcome situations likely to endanger life due to mechanical derangement. These are mostly obstructive in one way or another either to the organ itself, or to others around it. A cancer of the colon may block the intestinal conduit, as may cancers in the oesophagus, stomach and the rarer site of the small intestine. Intestinal obstruction gives rise to acute emergency since the condition itself is fatal if not corrected. Cancer is not by any means the sole cause of this condition; however, the numerous benign causes usually affect the small intestine which lies free in the abdomen hanging from a mesentery and is thus liable to snaring by a fibrous band or twist; whereas the large intestine for most of its course is plastered back on to the abdominal wall. As its name implies the large intestine has a larger bore; it also has a less muscular wall and does not ordinarily propel its contents as rapidly as the small intestine. Thus large bowel obstruction develops with less rapidity and less urgency. There are premonitory signs; small bowel obstruction, however, strikes with compelling urgency.

Whatever may be the chances of cure an operation is therefore often necessary for a bowel lesion in order either to avoid or overcome obstruction. There are other conditions requiring relief too, sometimes anaemia, sometimes diarrhoea. But obstruction is a paramount consideration elsewhere, in the brain (Chapter Five) and sometimes in the neck from the thyroid. The thyroid lies low in the neck; as it enlarges so it impinges upon the inlet to the chest. This is quite unyielding since the inlet is a bony girdle comprising ribs, vertebrae and breast bone. Through this inlet must pass amongst other things the oesophagus and the windpipe, the trachea. The thyroid is wrapped around the trachea so that its enlargement in its lower part, as it encroaches upon the thoracic inlet, takes place at the cost of the trachea with stifling effect. Not all thyroid growths do this but some may, just as many growths of the pancreas obstruct the bile duct which it envelops. Whereas relief of obstruction in the neck lies in removal of the thyroid by surgery or reduction of its size by X-rays, anatomy does not permit the ready removal of the pancreas – for the blood supply to the small intestine passes through it. So here relief cannot include removal of the organ and thus the possibility of cure. To overcome jaundice and damage to the liver the flow of bile has to be diverted at a higher level into the intestine without removal of the growth. In the lung the need for relief is less impelling for obstruction to one of the branches of the airway will not deprive the individual of so much respiratory function as to threaten life. However, incapacity may be enough to warrant treatment particularly if infection develops in the obstructed lung (Chapter Five).

Mechanical effects of a growth are rarely manifest in other ways. Only occasionally is removal of cancer in a limb necessary on account of the limitation it places on mobility. Ulceration is another matter; it is liable to bacterial contamination and infection, to cause a discharge and sometimes pain. For this reason a surface lesion may need to be removed whether or not it can be cured. Some growths lying beneath the skin, as in the breast, may develop outwards and fungate through the skin, a stage when eradication of the disease is unlikely but removal becomes necessary. Persistent bleeding must lead to anaemia and is prone to occur not from the gut alone but also from the urinary system calling for removal of the kidney or bladder or treatment with X-rays. Relief of symptoms or the avoidance and anticipation of serious complications perhaps provide the main objective of surgery and indeed of any other form of treatment – X-rays and cytotoxic drugs.

In addition an operation is often required to confirm the diagnosis. This is particularly true of the breast; simple swellings and cysts cannot always be recognized from cancer before being submitted to microscopic examination. The tumour has to be removed so that its nature can be ascertained, whether it is a cancer or not, and if it is, its degree of malignancy – so that an assessment of the future, the prognosis as we call it, can be made.

Symptoms, rather than presentation of a swelling, may give rise to the need for an exploratory operation. It is not always possible to be sure from examination of the patient or investigation what may be causing symptoms though the site of trouble may have been located within the chest or abdomen or elsewhere. Sometimes diagnostic X-rays reveal the shadow of a swelling or in the bowel the reverse, a stricture, demanding surgery if its nature is to be known.

Yet another need for operation arises in those cancers which are subject to hormonal influences. The female hormones, the oestrogens, appear to encourage cancer in the breast – not in all cases, but in many (Chapter Three). As already observed one approach lies in counteracting the hormonal influence. This can be achieved by an operation to remove the ovaries and adrenal glands, an operation which can be particularly effective in reducing seedlings resulting from dissemination, especially in bone. As an alternative, the pituitary, a ductless gland in the brain, which controls many if not most of the activities of the other ductless glands, is removed or destroyed. In the male counterpart the bone metastases of cancer of the prostate are also controllable by counteracting the male hormone either by removing the testes or by giving female hormones.

Surgery, then, fulfils a variety of functions in relation to cancer – diagnosis, relief of symptoms and, we hope, cure. It is a double-edged weapon since it may disturb the body's attempts at containment, and it is beginning to look as though these attempts are more successful than we had realized, that the disorder is often kept in check thereby for many years. However, operations will always be needed and until we have discovered means of boosting the natural defences the risk has to be accepted – the situation is no worse than it always has been for it has been accepted in ignorance in the past. It is rather different in relation to other forms of treatment such as X-rays and the use of cytotoxic drugs since they are given only on the premise of treatment either to relieve symptoms or cure.

Any chemical given by mouth or by injection which will destroy cells is cytotoxic. And, of course, these drugs if given in too large a dose will also kill. The aim is to find chemicals which are selective for any cancer; no useful purpose can be served by giving an oral dose of a substance known to destroy cancer cells if it is also likely to damage the sensitive cells which line the stomach and intestine. Nor can a drug be used which might be specific for a particular cancer if at the same time it destroys cells in the organ of its origin. Complete selectivity has not yet been achieved. The principle underlying the action of X-rays and cytotoxic drugs is that cancer cells are more sensitive than normal cells so that cancerous tissue will succumb to a dose which will not seriously or permanently affect the normal.

Unfortunately the white cells of the blood are, more than any other normal cells, sensitive to both irradiation and cytotoxic attack – though this holds in good stead when malignant conditions affecting these cells occur – the leukaemias and lymphoma (Hodgkin's disease). The most serious early effect of exposure to 'fall-out' from atomic explosion, which is radioactive and so causes irradiation, is the disappearance of white cells. Those who work in radioactive surroundings require routine blood tests to ensure that their white cells are not diminishing. And when applying cytotoxic drugs the white cell count is constantly monitored and not permitted to fall dangerously low, when resistance to infections ceases. By the same token the assault on cancer with these agents is also an attack upon the defences against it so that they suffer from a similar disadvantage as surgery; their effectiveness is limited by the paradox. We have no routine method of measuring the inhibition placed upon the lymphocytes though this is beginning to be possible on the research bench.

But while the approach to treatment may thus appear imprecise, as each year passes we are gaining more knowledge and treatment is gradually becoming more exact. With surgery this is less so partly because the lymphocytic effects are less well appreciated and partly because an operation can at best only be locally effective and must remain useless in terms of eradication when dissemination has occurred. This is true too of X-rays which are very accurately focused upon the cancer, but cannot be widely deployed. Cytotoxic drugs can be applied locally to an organ by introduction through its blood supply or by surface application. But our best hope for the future lies in the wider use of these drugs given in a way which ensures their distribution throughout the whole body.

CHAPTER EIGHT

The Effects of Treatment

Since operation in most circumstances denotes the removal of part or the whole of an organ it would be idle to suggest that treatment has no side effects. The same consideration applies to X-ray treatment in so far as it may destroy normal tissue outside the growth. Yet it is surprising how often a patient is unscathed by what was of necessity perpetrated upon him. If we look at this closer it becomes more understandable. Take the intestine for example. There is ample of it. Its function at the upper end is the secretion of enzymes so that its food may be broken down chemically and absorbed (Chapter Five). At the lower end it is chiefly concerned with the absorption of water. The internal lining which effects all this provides a greater area than the length of the intestine seen from outside would indicate. This is achieved through much folding of the lining within its muscular sheath. What has to be excised when a cancer of the bowel is removed is little compared with the total length, less still when compared with the lining which remains. So little function is lost, certainly too little to be noticeable.

Matters are less satisfactory if the growth is in the stomach; for this to be removed the greater part of the organ has to go. Moreover, the rearrangements necessary to restore continuity lead to a situation whereby the food bypasses the important duct from the pancreas and liver. So the chemicals in the bile and the enzymes from the pancreas which take part in digestion of the food escape their quarry, for it runs ahead of them. Instead of inter-mingling with the food as it passes by they have to catch up from behind a little later. At the same time the food itself is less well churned up and prepared, for the stomach is chiefly a pug-mill, designed to present to the gut beyond a homogeneous fluid bulk which will permit ready access for the digestive enzymes. With part of the stomach removed digestion is less perfect both in respect of pro-teins and fats. So after removal of part of the stomach a patient, though not subject to serious malnutrition is at least unlikely to gain weight; if the whole of the stomach is removed the effect is more severe. In addition, the indi-vidual is unable to eat large meals; he feels replete sooner. But this effect can be overcome by taking more frequent meals.

The blood itself can be affected in two ways by this operation. Iron is a substance necessary for the formation of the red pigment which carries the oxygen in the red blood cells. It is not readily absorbed in the gut partly because its compounds are at their most soluble in an acid medium and most of the intestine is alkaline. The stomach produces acid and iron is absorbed in that part of the intestine into which the food immediately passes from the stomach. This is the area which tends to get bypassed by the operation which has at the same time removed much of the stomach producing the acid. So anaemia may result with yet an additional adverse effect arising from the operation, for the stomach manufactures a special sub-stance in its lining which is taken up in the gut lower down and is responsible for the development of the red cell itself within the bone marrow. However, both these effects which dispose a patient to anaemia after partial or total removal of the stomach are readily overcome by giving the appropriate medicine. The individual must remain under permanent medical supervision after operation.

At the other end of the gut the disturbance and disability may clearly be greater. While it is sometimes possible to remove the final part of the gut – the rectum, in fact – and join up the ends so that natural voluntary control of bowel function by the final valve, known as the anus, is achieved, this is often impossible. In exchange for losing the growth and the unpleasant consequence that goes with it of bloody diarrhoea the patient has to accept a new opening on the front of the abdomen known as a colostomy. This is a daunting prospect, but incredible though it may seem to anyone facing it for the first time, once it has been established and its management mastered an individual with a colostomy can return to a normal and full life without social embarrassments.

It is not possible to construct a colostomy under the control of a new valve mechanism like the anus. Nevertheless it is brought under less direct and less obvious control; for the passage along the large intestine of its contents is regulated in part by the intake of food. It is usual for normal individuals to open their bowels in the morning either on getting up out of bed or after breakfast. This results from a conjunction of the start of normal daily activity and the reflex which causes intestinal contents to move onwards when more food is taken. That bowel irregularity exists is mainly because the exigencies of our daily life – the rush to get to work and so on – makes us fail to answer the natural urge to open the bowel instead of giving way to it. The rectum enables the stool to be retained and if this happens repeatedly constipation follows. There is much individual variation in this for some people need to open their bowels only once every other day or less frequently. It is only a convention that in normal healthy people the bowels will open at the same time each day, though this is true of the majority.

Once the rectum has been removed and a colostomy formed an impediment to regularity is removed. The bowels will move and can be trained to do so by leading a regular life as regards times of meals and sleeping so that with the aid of a cup of tea and for some (dare one mention it?) a smoke, the bowels will act soon after rising in the morning. Thereafter throughout the day the bowels will remain quiet, in some to act again in the evening, in others not until the next morning once more. Once the very natural revulsion to the prospect of such an unnatural opening has been overcome by adjustment to the idea and its management, the individual finds life not just manageable but fully so.

Common sense and a little reflection will indicate the consequences of surgery elsewhere. Removal of the womb for a growth of its outlet, the cervix, or the main part of the womb above, has usually to be undertaken after the menopause, so that there is no noticeable change. If before, then early artificial menopause is induced because the ovaries are usually removed as well. In this case hot flushes may persist as a cause of discomfort, but this is treatable by giving hormones. Fortunately the commonest tumour arising in the womb is the benign fibroid – not, therefore, a cancer – and for this only the tumour or the organ need be removed leaving the ovaries behind intact. But even after the removal of the ovaries a woman can still achieve an orgasm.

In man cancer of the testis affects one side so its removal does not lead to sterility. If the prostate has to go for cancer there, normal ejaculation is lost, though orgasm does occur.

When an organ is paired treatment of cancer is unlikely to have any consequences. Thus after the removal of one kidney the other has ample reserve to allow it to take over the job of two. Cancer in the urinary bladder is more

88

serious. This can be treated by forms of irradiation which leave the organ intact though it may become less distensible necessitating more frequent urination thereafter. If it has to be removed, a new small collecting reservoir is created from a section of the gut removed from intestinal circuit. Into this the pipes from the kidneys are placed. As in a colostomy no new voluntary control is possible and since urine is secreted fairly constantly it is necessary to collect it in a bag sealed to the skin and emptied when convenient. Such bags are slender and imperceptible under ordinary clothing.

Disfigurement is sometimes unavoidable but may be mitigated by numerous cosmetic devices. Nobody would deny that removal of a breast is a disfigurement. The consequences of this operation are less physical than psychological, since it infrequently happens before the end of the child-bearing period and the need for lactation. The psychological aspect causes a very real disturbance for which time is required to enable adjustment to be made, even though when the patient is dressed no evidence of removal of the breast is noticeable since an imitation is worn made to match the other side.

Limbs very seldom need to be amputated for cancer because the disease is rare in bone and muscle; and skin can be replaced readily by plastic surgery if cancer lies there. Artificial legs are so well designed that they function admirably and when the patient is clothed are unlikely to be perceived provided he or she trains himself to use the apparatus efficiently when walking. In this respect younger patients do better, for they are more adaptable. Since these rare cancers tend to occur earlier in life this is an important consideration.

It is surprising, too, how slight can be the effect of removal of a lung. The two lungs are contained on either side of the heart, its main vessels, the windpipe and the gullet, one lung filling in each side of the chest. Despite all these structures in between the two lungs, after the removal of one side the remaining lung can expand by pushing them over to the now empty side. The capacity of the remaining site is enough for daily living, though energetic exercise is precluded. In fact capacity is actually improved by removal of the affected lung which in its diseased state takes up space in the chest uselessly. This space is used to better purpose by the expansion of the remaining lung.

X-ray treatment is applied to cancers at any site either alone or in conjunction with surgery depending upon the nature and extent of the growth. Some cancers are resistant to the effects of X-rays, others particularly sensitive. In the latter case irradiation will be chosen in preference to operation, as it will where the tumour cannot reasonably be cut out either because of difficulty of access or because to do so would cause too much damage to vital tissue. This is true of many brain tumours. Normal nerve tissue is relatively impervious to X-rays, so that no damage is done to the brain by this form of treatment.

The immediate effect of any operation is weakening but paradoxically in the surgery of cancer this is often less noticeable than after an operation for a non-malignant disorder. This is because the presence of a growth can undermine the general health and its removal immediately allows correction and repair to get under way. It is rather different with X-ray treatment and cytotoxic drugs for these depress in a general way the activity of normal cells; so the patient recovers vigour and a feeling of well-being rather slowly over a matter of several weeks, even a month or two.

Thereafter life can be lived fully provided the individual has adjusted to new circumstances. Often the adjustment that is required is slight. Where it is greater its achievement is entirely a matter of personality. The achievement comes from within the individual, albeit supported and encouraged by doctors, nurses, family and friends. All the support they can give is quite ineffective without the will the individual can muster towards leading a normal life again.

CHAPTER NINE

Assessing the Results of Treatment

We are only on the verge of knowing what we are doing. After so many years of active treatment it should be possible to give clear answers regarding results, but it is not. Cancer registers have been set up and have long been in existence; much print has been pressed into a multitude of medical journals giving the results of treatment from innumerable centres and from individual doctors and this continues. A laudable competitiveness exists between groups in attempts to achieve ever better results, to show that variations of treatment or some new approach have been of benefit; to prove that efforts to encourage the patient to go to the doctor earlier to receive treatment increase the chances of cure. Nevertheless we are still in no position to be sure of the results. We often do not know whether our treatment changes events, nor in many instances do we know whether we can effect a cure. We place upon the sets of figures which have been impressed upon us a significance which critical examination must place in doubt. How can this be and how has our attention and concentration been so beguiled?

First there are the conventions which govern assessment. The yardstick for cancer statistics has always been the five-year 'cure'. It has been standard practice to follow cancer patients after operation, seeing them at regular intervals and 'scoring' survival after five-year intervals.

The percentage surviving from a group then represents the five-year cure rate – though humbler minds are now prone to speak of 'survival' rather than 'cure' rates for, the wish being father to the thought, some have been misled into believing that if five years pass without evidence of recurrence cure has been achieved. It is then possible to compare results between groups treated differently or treated similarly but by different individuals in different centres – or it should be.

But the convention is ill defined. It is understandable that in many surgical minds the climacteric moment of operation, the moment when the growth was removed, is the starting-point. But for comparative purposes this presents a flaw for the moment of treatment varies from one hospital to another and from patient to patient, and bears no constant relationship to the moment when the presence of the growth was revealed. Logically the onset of symptoms should represent the start of the quinquennium, but this also presents difficulties for it calls for an act of retrospection beyond the power of many patients. It can be very difficult to recall accurately when trouble began, if at all. Moreover, the symptom presenting the growth may be obscured by others which developed later and so are not directly relevant. The moment of diagnosis provides no better choice since diagnostic investigations may have to be pursued in some cases and not in others. So a compromise is reached: the date of first attendance at hospital at the time when the diagnosis was made is the official choice, but not so official as to be honoured more in the breach than the observance. And few reports actually state what date has been chosen. Thus true comparison is vitiated, though as the statistics of series begin to be handled in really large numbers by computers this will become less important – less important than the selection of cases which nullifies almost every surgical series published.

93

It is natural for a surgeon to review the cases he has operated upon and publish the five-year survival rate. He will probably divide them into those in whom it was found possible to remove all tissue suspected of harbouring growth and therefore with a reasonable chance of cure and those in whom only relief from the results of the growth was possible. In doing this he is making a double selection of a highly individualistic nature. His series will take no account of those who came to him but whom he did not consider fit for operation. Such a selection is inevitably personal for whereas one surgeon may regard operation in an advanced case not requiring relief as an interference unlikely to alter the course of the disease another may feel morally bound to make some attempt at removal, to take what chance there may be. Similar considerations apply to the positive selection between a curative procedure and an operation to relieve symptoms only. One surgeon will adopt a more aggressive approach than another. Nor are these considerations confined to surgical practice for the temperament of the physician in charge of X-ray treatment to a certain degree affects the dose of X-rays given or the regime of cytotoxic drugs prescribed.

But these are lesser flaws in the presentation of 'results', flaws which tend to be minimized when large numbers are considered so as to include results from numerous sources. Two fundamental problems remain and the first of these lies in our complete ignorance as to how long a patient may survive with an untreated growth. The effects of treatment of any disorder are properly assessed by comparing a group receiving treatment with a group which remains untreated; statistical analysis can then indicate whether a significant difference has been observed between the treated and the control group. This form of measurement is now common practice in medicine; new drugs, for example, are tested in this way. But it is clearly inhuman and unethical to deny treatment to a group of individuals suffering from a serious disease the effects of which it is thought may be mitigated by treatment and in which there is no clear indication that treatment is ineffectual. In cancer more than other diseases it has not been possible to withhold treatment from any group other than those in whom the possibility of cure is clearly out of the question. Nevertheless this group cannot serve as a control for comparison with those seen and treated for the disease at an earlier stage. In effect patients are treated and survival is assessed without collateral evidence of how long survival would have lasted if the disease had been left untreated. It could be that the progress of the cancer is unaltered by treatment; no firm evidence exists to the contrary.

The basic assumption that treatment effectively eliminates cancer bedevils the situation further. A not infrequent way of presenting results is to compare survival of groups treated at different stages of development of the same type of cancer. The stages of the disease on which assessment is achieved are mostly based on the findings when the patient is examined. Each stage provides evidence of spread of the disease. In the first stage evidence of cancer is confined to the primary growth itself. In the next either local lymph nodes are found to be involved or the primary tumour has spread beyond the original confines of its organ of origin and has begun to involve structures nearby, or both forms of spread may have occurred. The appearance of distant metastases represents the final stage. It is a relatively simple matter to 'stage' a growth near the surface from ordinary physical examination of the patient alone – as when the growth is in the breast. At less accessible sites such as the gut 'staging' can only be undertaken with accuracy from examination of the contents of the abdomen at the time of operation and from the specimen after it has been removed. Occasionally X-ray evidence may supply the information.

Staging, in effect, provides a breakdown of cases into groups based on clinical and pathological criteria in order to facilitate comparison at a later date between the stages. In this way different forms of treatment can be compared and their effectiveness assessed. Moreover, it can be seen whether a cancer responds to one form of treatment differently in a later stage compared with an earlier one.

The method is crude but it is the best we can devise at present. Clearly inaccuracies are inevitable. For example it may not be possible to perceive at examination an affected lymph node in the armpit of a fat patient with a cancer of the breast and though this may be picked up at operation other nodes carrying small deposits within them may escape notice even then and so never be produced for microscopic examination. Moreover, the very process of staging endorses and reinforces the notion that cancer is a disease of orderly progress, which it often is not. It takes no account of the possibility of dissemination at an early stage and the vagaries of malignant cell dissemination – that many cells fail to thrive while some may grow into metastases. The disorderliness of malignant spread together with the inevitable variation from one individual to another as regards immune response cannot be represented in such a system. The results must be vitiated thereby when small groups are compared. But variables thus introduced tend to lose significance as really large numbers are accumulated simply because the larger the series the nearer it approaches to the total population affected by that condition. The computer age enabling the handling and analysis of groups of tens of thousands rather than hundreds will improve our knowledge.

An example of how the system works is provided by

cancer of the rectum. This organ is not very clearly distinguished from the colon which leads into it; nobody, not the most expert anatomists, can tell us where colon ends and rectum begins. Suffice it to say that it is the last part of the gut and is about 15–17 cms. long. Its purpose is to inform us when our bowels need to be opened and provide information as to whether wind, fluid or solid is due to come out through the anus – the back passage, that is. Although its junction with colon is indistinct its other anatomical arrangements are such as to give clearer definition for the purpose of staging. The lymph drainage for the most part passes in one direction, as does the blood. Moreover, the blood runs through the special system provided for the gut into the liver; so malignant cells passing into the blood will be trapped in the liver and not at first be widely disseminated throughout the whole body. Thus one organ only, the liver, needs to be inspected in order to ascertain whether or not blood stream spread has occurred. Staging can be undertaken with fairer accuracy in the rectum than in almost any other organ, by examination at operation and examination of the specimen when it has been removed. Cancer of the rectum cannot however be classified into stages by examination of the patient; thus all cases not operated upon are excluded. The system can therefore only be applied as a measure of effectiveness of surgical treatment and, again, no comparison can be made with a group who have not been operated upon.

Of all patients with rectal cancer operated upon in whatever stage 55 per cent live to five years or beyond. In the first stage, with the cancer confined to the lining and not even invading the muscular coat of the bowel 85 per cent survive five years or more. When there is spread into muscle the figure becomes 67 per cent and beyond this 34 per cent. It is simple to deduce from this that the earlier the doctor sees a patient with cancer the better the chance of survival. This may, however, be fallacious.

In the first place seeing the doctor early implies seeing him as soon as symptoms are observed by the patient and this is a very different thing from 'early' in terms of the growth. The growth may be early. Alternatively it may have developed unnoticed by the patient for years and so be late or it may have disseminated at an early stage. In short, symptoms do not correlate with the progress of the disease and do not reflect the stage it has reached. This is borne out by another statistic.

Of all patients presenting who are operated upon for rectal cancer 15 per cent are found to be in the first stage: that is with the cancer confined to the lining of the organ and with an 85 per cent chance of living beyond five years. The strange fact is that this proportion of 15 per cent in the best group has remained the same in this country for at least forty years. Many changes have taken place in our social structure during that time, including the advent of the health service so that medical services have become more readily available and hospital facilities more accessible. There is no doubt that patients are now seeking medical care earlier, in terms of their symptoms, than they did years ago. And yet the proportion of 'early' cases in terms of the growth itself has remained the same. If symptoms reflected the progress of the growth and if that progress took place in orderly fashion, then we could properly expect an increased number of patients to be seen at the first stage.

This figure of 15 per cent is universal in all countries from which comparable figures can be obtained as is its persistence unchanged over the last few decades. The explanation for it must partly lie in the fact that symptoms and the progress of the diseases do not match; it also indicates the variability in any one type of cancer, the conglomerate nature of its different forms. One case is not the same as another for one may be mild and slowly progressive in orderly fashion, while another becomes disorderly and progressive at any early stage of its existence. That 15 per cent must represent the proportion within the group of rectal cancers as a whole which is more benign and therefore likely to give rise to long survival; it is not the progenitor group of those seen for the first time in stage two though it is likely to reach the second stage later in its existence – long after it has declared itself by its symptoms. In support of this is an observation relating to the large bowel as a whole, of which the rectum is just an integral part.

Symptoms are noticed in patients for variable periods before they seek advice. In medical terminology the 'history' – that is the account of the symptoms up to the moment the patient is seen by the doctor – may be long or short. Surprisingly the longer the history in large bowel cancer the longer the ultimate survival. While this is yet another clear demonstration that the 'early' case cannot be correlated with early development of the cancer, it still remains to be explained why one group of patients will allow their symptoms to persist longer and why this should prove to be those with a better outlook. Individuality being what it is, it is quite understandable that there would be variability – that one person for one reason or another will put up with what disturbs him for longer than his neighbour. But the correlation with longer survival vitiates any explanation on grounds of the personality or circumstances of the individual. It can only mean that here is a species of large bowel cancer which is different. It remains limited to its primary site for many years and does not grow or extend as other large bowel cancers do in a way that causes them to induce more compelling symptoms such as colic from partial blockage. Just like the skin, in fact. Here we are able to see that the rodent ulcer (Chapter Four) is different from other skin cancers. Nobody considers this to be the first stage of the others; it is an entity to itself even though it is a skin cancer. And so it may be with stage one of rectal cancers; if, as it seems, this is so staging as a means of assessment is open to many doubts, not only in the large bowel but elsewhere in the body.

It must be emphasized that survival figures attempt to reflect two main factors. One is our ability to overcome the side effects of a growth, be it an ulcer or a tumour, which may lead to sickness and possibly death through obstruction, bleeding and the like. The other is eradication of cancer. The two are very different. Clearly treatment is effective in prolonging survival (not to mention improvement of the quality of life which is unquantifiable) by the removal of growths which in some way, usually mechanically, disturb function of the organ they arise in. If no case of bowel cancer was operated upon many patients would die the sooner from obstruction. There can be no question therefore that the methods of treatment we have today are necessary, and effective in improving survival.

But eradication of the disease is another matter. Survival figures give no indication that this is achieved. Misunderstanding and even confusion have been caused by the presentation of the two effects of treatment, the one palliative (that is relief) the other eradicative, in the one set of statistics. But it cannot be otherwise since treatment at one and the same time is an attempt to achieve both objectives. At least in most cancers. There is one site of cancer, however, where survival is coterminous with the growth itself, where the growth as it develops does not bring in its wake malfunction in a vital organ. That is the breast. Death, when it occurs due to breast cancer, is always at a late stage and due to wide spread.

Breast cancer is staged on the basis of findings at examination of the patient. A correction can be made at operation. This used to be more possible than now, for until recently surgical extirpation demanded clearance of all the lymph nodes in the armpit and these could then be examined for evidence of growth. Now operation is often limited to removal of the breast alone for it has been found that survival is better if lymph nodes are not removed or subjected to X-rays – a further indication that the lymphatic cells are to be encouraged (Chapter Six). Since it is based on physical examination breast staging is therefore subject to observer error. But if we accept this, and errors tend to rule one another out as large numbers are considered, the evidence from breast staging can be taken as a model of the effects of treatment on eradication of the cancer alone.

Staging of breast cancer is in principle the same as elsewhere with slight variations considered to indicate yet another step in the process of spread, as for example the attachment of the growth to the skin or the muscle on which the breast lies. The survival of cases is presented graphically by plotting the percentage who survive annually, thus producing a falling curve. Separate graphs are made for each stage and these demonstrate clearly enough that the survival rate is better for stage one than stage two and so on. So far so good, and you might think that here is evidence that earlier treatment results in longer survival. But the system takes no account of the duration of the disease; it is concerned only with what may be expected of treatment at a certain stage. It is a mistake to believe that we can draw conclusions that the course of the disease has been altered.

Let us try to look at this from the aspect of the natural progress of the cancer itself – the life of the cancer rather than of the patient – and consider what the graph of the mean survival of all patients would look like from the time their growths started rather than when they presented for treatment. Again we should get a curve. If only we knew when a growth actually started – and more about this in the next chapter – it is likely that the first part of the graph would be a straight horizontal line indicating survival for many years; in all probability cancers take a long time before they make themselves felt. After this the line would be a curve downwards and this curve would resemble the summation of our previous curves for the various stages put together end on successively.

Perhaps this is a difficult concept and it can be grasped in another way. The survival rate is less for those in stage two than stage one. But at stage two the disease has progressed farther than stage one. It is later in terms of the cancer than at stage one when patients would in any case survive longer and are therefore represented at a higher and flatter part of the curve. The stage two patients have already, in respect of their cancer, had part of their survival time before they were seen. In other words, for stage two cases to be diagnosed in stage one we should be operating on them last year and not this. Their time of survival from operation would then be longer, but there is no proof that their survival from the start of the growth would be any greater. In terms of the cancer we would not have altered its course. The patient in stage two has simply had longer with the disease before operation and less time afterwards and operation may have been an intervention of no significance.

All that this serves to demonstrate is that staging has limited application. The effects of different forms of treatment can be examined by comparison within one stage, but not between two different stages. Perhaps a glimpse of the obvious but it has a corollary. It is an understandable axiom of cancer education and propaganda that patients should be seen earlier for treatment would then have a better chance of success: that is, it would be followed by better results in terms of survival. Indeed it would, but the success relates more to the state of development of the cancer than the effectiveness of the treatment. The misconception arises here from an unconscious comparison of treatment between two stages, of comparing like with unlike.

This is not to say that patients should neglect symptoms which might be due to cancer. The earlier they are seen the better, to eliminate the side effects. But we have no means of judging the effects of treatment in terms of the elimination of all cancer cells within the body. Survival may be prolonged but cells remain either to recur at the original site or to appear as metastases at a later date.

There are so many imponderables. We do not know how long an interval elapses between the onset of a cancer and death for there is no way of knowing when it started. It is obvious that some cancers do not lead to death and these are not confined to certain restricted sites; the nature of the malignant cell and the immunological reaction in each individual case are the components which dictate this. No terms of reference or means of measurement have yet been devised to render these components registerable and make comparison between one group and another possible. This and our inability to know whether or not dissemination has already occurred when a patient is first seen not only limits prediction in the individual patient – prognosis, that is – but also denies us the ability to see cancer in the wider sense of its natural history in any population and makes the assessment of overall results difficult.

Above all, there are as yet no techniques by which a cancer can be observed at its outset, no way of discerning the change of normal cells into a new generation of malignancy cells. Until this can be done it will not be possible to compute with any accuracy the duration of the disease in its many forms, nor true survival. This knowledge will come; for if we think of looking for it the means will be found – and this is just one aim which has been obscured by the emotive appeal for the 'early' case of current orthodoxy. When it does come many may be surprised to discover how long the disorder remains discreetly hidden.

All that has been said relates to results in general, to general statistics. To say that there is no statistical evidence to indicate that treatment can eliminate all cancer cells in the body and thus effect a complete cure is not to say that an individual case is not cured. Indeed the vast majority of common skin cancers are cured, the growth is removed and does not recur, but in most forms this is not a lethal condition even untreated. There is no doubt other growths which could prove lethal are sometimes seen and treated before cell dissemination has occurred. These are potentially curable. Disseminative growth is not necessarily a serious sentence; many years can elapse before distant cellular seedlings begin to make their presence felt – twenty or more. There are numerous examples of survival beyond five years in patients with large bowel cancer in whom secondary growth was present in the liver at the time they were first seen. Certain forms of chronic leukaemia in the elderly can be allowed to go untreated since they do not kill. Though at some sites the course of cancer may be brief, as in the gullet where survival periods have to be reckoned in two rather than five years, taken all over the disease is not the quick killer nor the painful sentence many would suppose.

It would be quite wrong to conclude that no improvement has been achieved. A general steady improvement in length and quality of survival has taken place overall since the beginning of the century even if complete elimination of the disease still escapes us. There is much evidence of a considerable increase in the number of patients who can now be made fit to undergo treatment due to the introduction of antibiotics to deal with infection, improvements in blood transfusion and other measures. Thus of every 100 patients now presenting with cancer of the large bowel 95 undergo operation compared with 45 forty years ago. This is a considerable gain as regards lengthened survival measured in five-year terms and in early mortality, since fewer patients die from the effects of obstruction, anaemia and infection. Moreover, the quality of life is improved for many thereby. Nevertheless the overall survival (that is those treated with the hope of cure taken together with those who are not), for all cases of large bowel cancer has not changed during the last decade or more. The improved operation rate has therefore not impinged upon the overall figures for survival. This statistic remains unaltered as another indication that the spread of the disease has already been determined by the time it declares itself; that with the means which have been at our disposal we cannot detect the truly early case at a stage when elimination of all cancer cells is a possibility.

At the present time cancer treatment appears to have reached a culmination, a peak beyond which we have not moved for several decades. But there are more than signs that we are about to make a leap forward.

CHAPTER TEN

The Future

The future looks hopeful, more so than for many years if only because scepticism has now begun to remove the blinkers which for so long maintained blind faith in removal by any means, to the exclusion of sophistication. A new evaluation is taking place for numerous reasons. The awareness that blood stream dissemination possibly takes place early in the life of a growth and may even be more than sporadic has reinforced our belief, hitherto rather tenuously held, that numerous factors militate against the malignant cells; for the number of distant seedlings which become manifest is infinitely few compared with the showers of cells which must be released from the primary growth. Furthermore, the cells which survive to become seedlings can lie dormant for a considerable time. So it has become evident that there are processes of reaction and that treatment would be more effective if aimed at enhancing them. Certainly the methods now in use should be re-evaluated with in mind the avoidance of anything which may inhibit the reaction of normal tissues to invasion. It has recently come to light that some growths can even revert to normal; the derangement of the nuclei which produced the malignant cells can switch back to normal form. Though this reversion is a rare event only seen so far in a few unusual tumours it provides another reason for avoiding too energetic use of forms of treatment which in themselves disturb nuclear material, such as irradiation.

The period between the birth of the first generation of a malignant cell line and their manifestation as a detectable growth is unknown. Clearly it is important to know more about the silent period between the start of the cancer and its manifestation. Is this long or brief? For if it is long this should give an opportunity to seek and detect it and perhaps to destroy it before it has broken loose and spread. Mathematical models can be constructed to indicate the length of time one malignant cell would take to grow to a tumour. In leukaemia it is sometimes possible to conclude from the similar identity of all the circulating malignant cells that the disease started originally from one cell firing off into malignancy. However, there is no certainty that this is true of all tumours. Such models must therefore be seen as an indication. Nor do they take into account the restraining effects of the immune reactions which vary not only from individual to individual but probably from time to time in any one person. Nevertheless it is worth a glance at such a system despite its imperfections.

It is reasonable to accept the average size of a malignant cell as 10 microns – about the same as a red cell (Chapter Two). If the time it takes for a malignant cell to reproduce to two cells – the doubling times – is a hundred days by the end of a year the malignancy will not have reached its fourth division. Its continued growth at a steady rate by geometrical progression will produce a tumour of a billion cells by ten years and only then will have a diameter of one centimetre. One centimetre is about the size of a tumour which can just be felt in the breast. Two more years will see it at four centimetres. This doubling time is arbitrary. However, it is possible to measure a palpable tumour in the breast and, if for some reason it is not removed, its rate of increase in size can be measured and the doubling time of the cells contained in it can be estimated. This form of analysis, though inaccurate for many reasons, shows variability as might be expected. Some tumours grow slowly with a cell doubling time of 450 days; at the other end of the scale they increase with a doubling time of 90 days. If we then try to look backwards to the moment when the growths started from one cell we find that it must have taken forty-two and eight years respectively for the cancers to reach presentable size. In a particular study the beginning of these periods roughly coincided with puberty and menopause.

There is much speculation in this; cell division and with it tumour growth probably fluctuates. It may advance suddenly or may be held or even turned back at stages in the life of the cancer by variations in the potency of the immunological response. Nevertheless the exercise indicates, at least, that cancer cells may be present for a very considerable time before a tumour develops of size sufficient to be felt. Here may be a chance for intervention before cell dissemination. It might prove possible to detect the presence of cancer cells and the means whereby this could be done are dimly discernible now. Cancers produce biochemical effects by disturbing the complex composition of the proteins in the blood. This may in part be a reflection of the immunological response since antibodies are attached to proteins and with modern sophisticated methods of analysis there is increasing evidence that antibodies, for so long thought to be held in abeyance in this disease (Chapter Six), are in fact produced – in particular against melanoma, one of the skin cancers (Chapter Three). The search is now on for antibodies to other cancers – the more so because it has been known for some time that one form of mucus secreting cancer in the bowel can provoke weak antibodies. As more become demonstrable these in themselves could be used as an indicator of the presence of cancer cells. Whether they are present and in sufficient quantity for detection in the phase before a growth is ordinarily diagnosible remains to be seen.

Meanwhile detection in the clinical phase is improving. The 'cervical smear' which has led to the measures for the prevention of uterine cancer is an obvious case in point. The uterine cervix is a common site for cancer; here it is possible to detect malignant cells and, better, cells which appear to be changing towards malignancy but are not yet invasive. A scraping from the cervix removes sufficient of the latter for identification under the microscope. At this early stage removal of the cervix alone may prevent cancer though as yet there is no statistical evidence to indicate a reduction in the incidence of cervical cancer as a result of the procedure. *Cancer-in-situ*, as this stage is called, can also be seen not infrequently in the prostate. This gland has to be removed when it enlarges as it often does in later age causing an obstruction to urinary outflow from the bladder. In such prostates, which have become enlarged through a process not due to cancer, individual *cancer-in-situ* cells are sometimes seen. Although the prostate is not as readily accessible as the cervix so that preventive investigation at special clinics is not yet a practical proposition, a method of obtaining a biopsy specimen by inserting a needle is now developing.

Longstanding inflammation disposes towards malignant change. A potent though not common example of this lies in the intestine. After ten years inflammatory disease of the large intestine, colitis, carries a high risk of cancer – thirty times higher with a mean age for presentation twenty years earlier than in individuals without colitis. It is difficult to detect such change for the warning symptoms, bleeding and diarrhoea, are identical with those of the original disease. Nor is it readily demonstrated by X-rays as is cancer developing in normal bowel. Since this malignant change does not appear to disseminate early this cancer is one of those amenable to cure if the bowel is removed in the early stages. The danger lies in missing the early stage. Recently, alteration in the appearances of the lining cells of the bowel affected by colitis has been noticed, which though not actually depicting malignancy is a warning of impending malignant change.

Mass radiography whereby whole communities can be screened by diagnostic chest X-rays is more of a public health than a preventive measure, for this can only reveal diseases which have started but not yet given rise to symptoms and so have not been suspected. One of these diseases is cancer, but in this instance a fully developed growth is revealed and no evidence is forthcoming that the survival statistics of lung cancer have been altered by mass radiography.

Detection of cancer at an earlier stage is one thing. If this becomes possible by biochemical means – a sample of blood showing a change in the normal pattern of proteins for example – it will give rise to another problem: how to locate the cancer. For it is the intent of earlier detection to indicate the presence of cancer at a stage before it is manifest through the ordinary means of diagnosis in use today. The growth will be too small to be seen, felt or displayed by diagnostic X-rays. So chemical means of destroying malignant cells will increase in importance.

The cytotoxic drugs act on the malignant cell in two ways. There are what are known as the alkylating agents which bind themselves to the D.N.A. of the malignant cell nucleus (Chapter Two) and so alter it that it becomes ineffective. It is thus denied the opportunity of reproducing itself and further malignant cells cannot form. The alternative mechanism strikes at the processes whereby D.N.A. can be formed. The drugs which achieve this are antimetabolites. Metabolism is the process of building up living matter from amino-acids, which create protein, and from other materials. The antimetabolites interfere with the pathways by which the metabolism of the malignant nucleus is conducted with the result that the D.N.A. cannot increase.

Cytotoxic drugs are in their infancy. Nevertheless they have already begun to show remarkable results in cancer of the circulating white cells (Chapter Three). One particular form of this, acute lymphoblastic leukaemia, affects babies and young children. There has been no effective treatment hitherto so the average survival time is known. It is three to five months. This average has now increased to three years and there are some children who are living considerably longer than this. To achieve this requires the use of both alkylating agents and antimetabolites given one after the other for it has been found that the continuous use of one cytotoxic drug is effective for a while and then fails. The reason for this is the extraordinary ability of nuclear material to adapt. Thus many but not all the malignant cells are destroyed by one drug. Some can resist its effect and then grow to provide a new generation of resistant cells. At this stage another drug with a different mechanism of cytotoxic effect can be brought into action. Thus different drugs are given in succession at intervals – a 'pulse' effect. And here a knowledge of the doubling time of the malignant cell is of importance for it is clearly advantageous to give a new drug at the time when a new generation of malignant cells is expected to be born from those which resisted the previous drug.

Obviously ingenuity and sophistication are required for the effective use of these drugs, based on knowledge and experience which are gradually being gained and which should widen their scope. One antimetabolite has been discovered of unusual promise. All cells need a substance, asparagine; normal cells are capable of producing this for themselves, but malignant cells are not. So the malignant cells have to rely upon what may be had from the normal cells around them. If this supply could be denied to them they should cease to flourish and wither away. It so happens that some bacteria develop an enzyme (Chapter Five) asparaginase which destroys asparagine. This can be extracted from bacterial cultures. So here is a substance which will put a stop to malignant cells but will not impede the replication of normal cells. In comparison cytotoxic drugs are less specific. It has, however, some disadvantages which have tarnished its early promise. Though it cures experimental tumours in mice, man is more sensitive to the general toxic effects of the drug. It has proved useful for acute leukaemia. As to its more general use there is one more serious disadvantage, it suppresses the immunity response (Chapter Six).

Immunity holds great hopes for the future and ingenuity has been no less in this field. There have been straightforward approaches such as stimulating the immunological mechanisms by injecting vaccines containing killed bacteria or their toxins which have been so altered as not to poison the individual. But this invokes the antibody reaction which plays a lesser part in the immunity to cancer than the lymphocyte (Chapter Six). The thought lying behind this is the hope that both systems will be encouraged.

Rather more subtle is the use of viruses – setting a thief to catch a thief since viruses are one of the factors responsible for causing cancer. There are an infinite variety of viruses; some alter the nucleus of normal cells so that they become cancerous (Chapter Two); others attack cells and destroy them. Attempts have been made to find or develop a virus which will destroy a malignant cell in preference to a normal one. This has been successful in animal experiments but less so in man. Less directly, that is, for by introducing viruses in man – cancers have been injected with smallpox vaccine for example – immunity is again invoked. So although some beneficial effects have been noted they usually are transient.

Ingenious developments are taking place in cell biology. Recently cells taken from cancers in mice have been united with normal cells from the same animal. They are fused together to form another living cell, the nucleus of which is part malignant, part normal. This is a hybrid, like a mule, which is the offspring of a horse and an ass. As a result of the conjunction malignancy is lost; the hybrid cell is not malignant. So the next step is to develop hybrids to human cancer cells. This will be a complex matter. First cells from the cancer will have to be grown outside the body in a special culture, then put alongside normal cells from the same individual and fused together by the action of a virus. From that point it is difficult to foresee how this discovery could be applied for to return these to the patient would only be to return cells no longer malignant and they would not start a chain reaction of hybridization in the cancer cells still in the patient's body. Alternatively it might eventually prove possible to introduce a virus to the patient to bring about the cell fusion there, but this is most improbable and would be very likely to have dangerous side effects.

A more promising approach is the formation of hybrids between malignant cells in man and non-malignant cells from another species for the latter should invoke graft rejection (Chapter Six) when the combination is returned to the patient. In this case the hybrid cells could create a chain reaction for they would call into action the immunological forces of the patient's lymphocytes. Mice have been immunized in this way by hybrids from mouse cancer and normal cells from hamster.

Much is therefore being done in the laboratory. It is no coincidence that the first real prospects of effective elimination of cancer, not by preventing the disease but as it arises in the individual, are appearing at a time when man has learnt how to manipulate his own cells in a number of frightening ways, not least how to fertilize an ovum outside the body with the possibility of replacing it for growth into a pre-designed being. Human engineering has sinister undertones but it will open doors to the solutions we aspire to for cancer. These may be achieved soon, in the next ten years perhaps. Understanding of the nature of cancer and the integral and inevitable part it plays in life and living on this planet will provide a spur to the application of the new discoveries.

Appendix

In order to give some idea of the incidence of cancer this selected list of figures has been taken from the Registrar General's statistics for England and Wales. Some guidance and explanation is needed.

A comparison of deaths with the total population reveals the annual death rate from cancer to be only slightly greater than 2 per cent.

It should be understood that these figures only provide indications of trends; no firm deductions can be drawn. For example the total population increased by approximately 3,500,000 during the period; the increase in deaths from cancer over the period was relatively greater. But it cannot be assumed from this that cancer is on the increase generally. It would be necessary to refer to a breakdown of age-groups since the increase in population might be due to a general trend to longer survival with a more aged population. This would be likely to create a bias due to cancer being more prevalent in old age-groups. Conversely, the actual fall in incidence in those cancers with a declining trend may be greater than appears.

A glance down the columns immediately discloses the commoner sites of the disease.

Under the year 1964 there are two columns of figures. The first is for new cases registered – 1964 is the last year for which such figures are available. Against them are the deaths from cancer in the same year for the same sites. Although most of the deaths clearly did not occur in the new cases registered for that year, the death rate of cancer at most sites has remained approximately the same throughout the decade preceding 1968, the last year for which mortality figures are at present available. There are some notable exceptions; the mortality for carcinoma of the bronchus and breast has risen reflecting the increasing incidence of these diseases. The situation is reversed at other sites with a falling incidence in uterine cancer and possibly in skin. Comparing cases registered and deaths in 1964 the figures for skin cancer demonstrate its unlethal nature and for breast cancer indicate that there may be a group who do not succumb.

	1958	1964	1964	1968
Total population England and Wales	45,109,000		47,344,300	48,593,000
	Deaths	New cases	Deaths	Deaths
All malignancies	97,000	141,070	106,194	113,936
Mouth and Pharynx	1,924	3,498	1,676	1,653
Lip	82	619	62	66
Tongue	500	559	427	351
Oesophagus	2,295	2,478	2,541	2,901
Stomach	14,112	11,236	13,069	12,749
Colon	9,378	9,892	9,300	9,943
Rectum and Recto-Sigmoid Junction	5,607	7,289	5,540	5,890
Bronchus and Lung	19,718	29,994	25,247	28,782
Breast	9,029	16,169	9,919	10,280
Uterine Cervix	2,689	5,301	2,566	2,434
Uterus	1,413	3,434	1,412	1,537
Prostate	3,614	5,132	3,730	3,939
Testis	204	527	220	256
Bladder	2,849	5,537	3,355	3,697
Skin	480	14,303	425	428
Melanoma of Skin	353	920	479	527
Brain and Nervous System	1,856	2,405	1,966	1,897
Bone	637	456	504	559
Leukaemia	2,386	2,863	2,867	2,729

Glossary

ADRENAL   A hormone-secreting gland responsible for growth and reactions to stress.

ALVEOLI   The individual sac-like chambers of the lungs where oxygen transfer takes place between inspired air and the blood.

ANDROGENS   Male hormones.

ANEUPLOIDY   An increase in the nuclear content of a cell by a partial increase in chromosomes as opposed to additional full sets of chromosomes as in polyploid cells (see polyploidy).

ANTIBIOTICS   Chemicals which kill bacteria in the body.

BRONCHUS, BRONCHI   The main air tubes from the windpipe (trachea) into the lungs.

CAPILLARIES   Minute blood vessels at the end of the arterial supply and the beginning of the venous drainage.

CHROMOSOMES   The filamentous units of a cell nucleus which by their number identify the species and by the composition endow the individual with his personal characteristics. Biochemically they are composed of D.N.A. which sets the cellular pattern of work. Thus the species and individual characteristics are stamped upon cellular activity.

CIRRHOSIS   An abnormal condition of the liver which may follow damage due to various causes such as infections and poisoning (with alcohol for example).

COLOSTOMY   An artificial opening from the colon onto the front of the abdomen.

CYTOPLASM   The cell is a unit comprising a nucleus which dictates and regulates the work of the cell. This floats in the cytoplasm, which is in effect a nondescript material in which the biochemical activities of the cell ordained by the nucleus can be carried out. The cytoplasm and the nucleus are contained within a sack – the cell membrane.

CYTOTOXIC DRUGS   Drugs which inhibit or kill cells in the body.

DESOXYRIBONUCLEIC ACID (D.N.A.)   The chemical which forms the nucleus and initiates and controls cell function. It is also responsible for cell reproduction.

DUODENUM   The uppermost part of the intestine into which the stomach empties.

ECTODERM   The outer ensheathing layer of cells which develop as the ovum grows and eventually become the surface cells of the skin, the lining cells of the gut, lungs, urinary tract, etc. The ball of cells which constitutes the growing ovum folds onto itself, or invaginates, as will a rubber ball when it is collapsed. The ensheathing cells which remain outside are the ectoderm which gives rise to the skin and any glands associated with it, such as sweat gland and the breast; the nerves also arise from ectoderm. Those ensheathing cells which get turned in, the endoderm, provide the lining of the gut and any glands associated with that.

EMBRYO   The early stage of the developing baby in the womb.

119

ENDODERM   See ectoderm.

ENDOPLASMIC RETICULUM   The ducting system within cell cytoplasm which allows the chemical product of the cell to be collected and exported from the cell.

ENZYME   A secretion which activates a biochemical reaction as in the process of digestion.

EPITHELIAL CELLS   The cells of the surfaces of skin and gut, and in the lungs, urinary tract, etc.

EPITHELIUM   The layer of cells which provide the surface of the skin and of the inner lining of hollow organs or tubes. It is derived from ecto- or endoderm.

GAMETE   The reproductive particles – either the ovum before fertilization or the sperm.

HAEMOGLOBIN   The chemical in the red blood cell responsible for oxygen transport. It is a pigment and gives the blood, through its individual cells, its colour.

HOMINID   That part of the human family evolutionarily related to and including man.

HORMONE   A chemical messenger created in one cell to activate function in another.

LUMEN   The space, or potential space, within a tube such as the gut; the channel of a biological ducting system.

LYMPHATICS   The fine pipes which carry the tissue fluid, which is lymph, and lymphatic cells back to lymph glands and eventually back to the blood stream.

LYMPHOCYTE   One of the main white cells of the blood concerned with immunity.

MESENTERY   The sling of peritoneum which attaches the intestine to the back of the abdominal cavity.

MESODERM, MESOTHELIUM   As the ovum grows it forms an accumulation of cells. The outer layer eventually become the cells on all surfaces – the skin, the lining of the gut, of the lungs, etc., and the nerves. The inner cells, the mesoderm, give rise to all supporting structures – the bones, muscles, connective tissue and the blood cells. See also ectoderm.

METABOLISM   The whole function of energy production and utilization in biology.

METASTASES   Growing seedlings at sites remote from the original growth, detectable on examination of the patient or by investigation.

MICRON   The unit of measurement used in microscopy; one millionth part of a metre.

MORPHOLOGY   The shape; or the study and science of shape and form.

MUCOSA MUCOUS MEMBRANE   The secretory inner lining of hollow organs such as the gut. Epithelial cells provide the surface and the small glands in its substance, which include mucus secreting glands.

NECROTIC   Necrosis is death of tissue or cells; hence necrotic.

OESTROGENS   Female hormones.

PATHOLOGICAL   Abnormality of cell or tissue form and function.

PERIOSTEUM   The membrane in which bone is ensheathed.

PERITONEUM   The smooth lining to the abdominal cavity.

PLEURA   The smooth lining within the cavity of the chest and over the surface of the lungs.

POLYPLOIDY   An increase in nuclear content of a cell

due to a direct multiple of the normal complement of chromosomes.

PROGNOSIS   The outlook.

REPLICATION   To replicate is to reproduce so as to replace in contradistinction to reproduction in order to multiply.

RIBONUCLEIC ACID (R.N.A.)   The chemical in the cell which carries out the instruction of the D.N.A. of the cell nucleus. (See D.N.A.)

SEBUM   A protective secretion from glands in the skin maintaining the skin's texture (natural Nivea).

SENESCENCE   Ageing and the changes that go with it.

SOMATIC   The soma denotes the physical element of the body. Somatic is the adjective – hence somatic cells, a term used to distinguish all those tissues of the body outside the brain and nervous system.

SYNOVIA   The smooth inner lining of a joint.

TOTIPOTENTIAL CELL   Having the ability to develop into every form of cell and thus provide every tissue.

VIRUS   A class of infective agent smaller than a bacterium. It is smaller than a cell and is virtually a particle of nucleoprotein.